PLANT-BASED COOKING

50 Green Recipes Focused on Natural Food, Using Everyday Ingredients That Will Work Wonders on Your Well-Being

Botanika Green Way

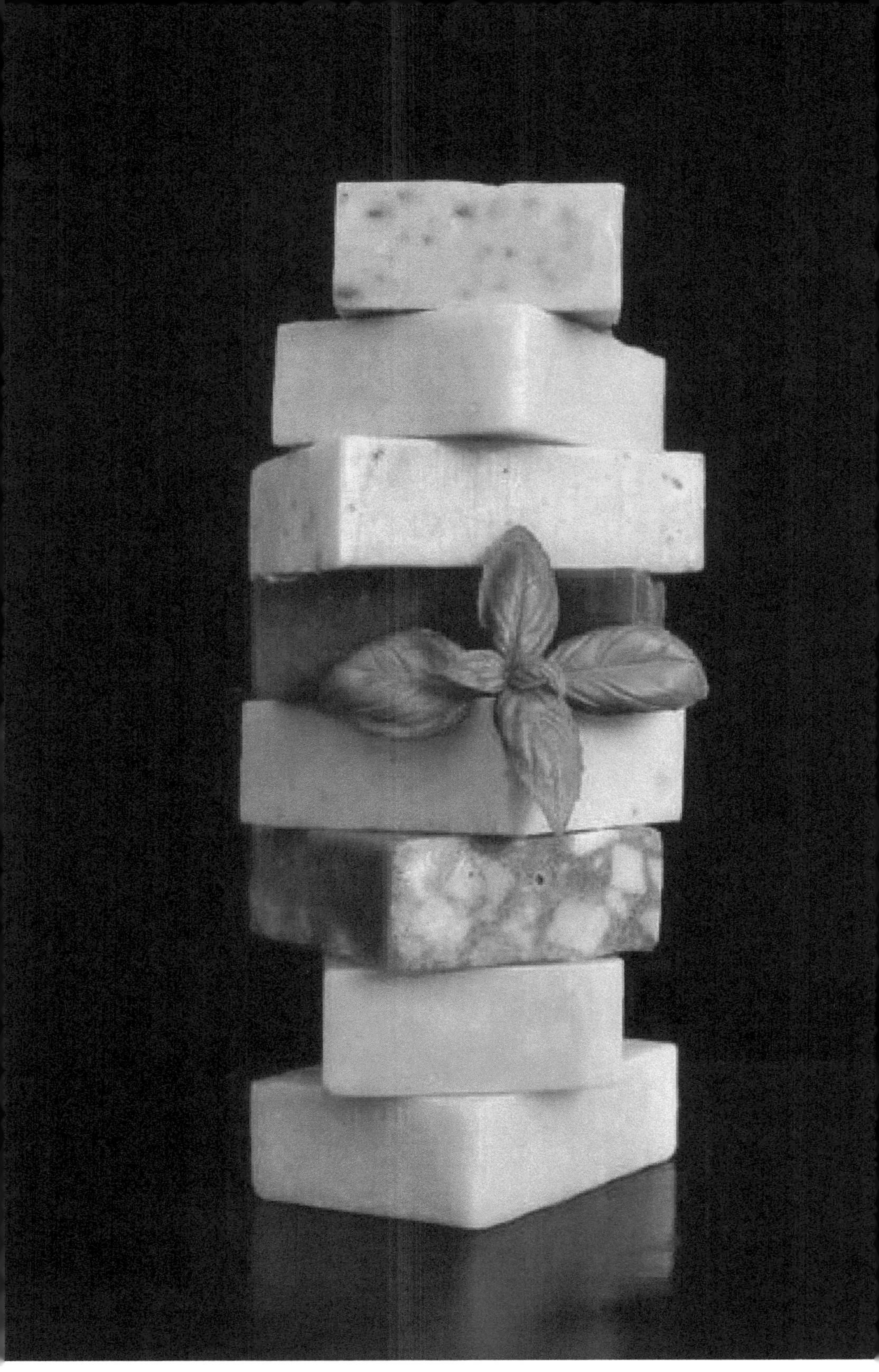

liable for any hardship or damages that may befall them after undertaking the information described herein.

Additionally, the information in the following pages is intended only for informational purposes and should thus be thought of as universal. As befitting its nature, it is presented without assurance regarding its prolonged validity or interim quality. Trademarks that are mentioned are done without written consent and can in no way be considered an endorsement from the trademark holder.

Table of Contents

INTRODUCTION

A plant-based diet is a diet based primarily on whole plant foods. Hence, it excludes animal-sourced foods, hydrogenated oils, refined sugars, and processed foods. A whole food plant-based diet does not consist solely of fruits and vegetables. It includes unprocessed or barely processed oils with healthy fats like extra-virgin olive oil, whole grains, legumes, seeds, and nuts, as well as herbs and spices.

What is the Plant-Based Diet?

The plant-based diet may seem similar to a vegetarian or vegan diet, but it is neither. It's not a diet but a healthy lifestyle. It uses food from plants, and it excludes processed foods like white rice and added sugars, which are allowed in vegan and vegetarian diets.

A plant-based diet is not a diet; it's a healthy way of life

The secret to a healthy diet is simpler than you ever thought! When following a plant-based dietary regimen, you should focus on plant-based foods and avoid animal-sourced food. Whether you are already following a vegan diet or are considering trying this lifestyle, this plant-based, budget-friendly food list makes your grocery shopping easy to manage.

- **VEGETABLES**

Try to include different types of vegetables in your diet from above-ground vegetables to root vegetables, which grow underground.

- **FRUITS**

Choose affordable fruits that are in season. Add frozen fruit to your grocery list since they are just as nutritious as fresh produce. They can be used in smoothies, toppings, compotes, or preserves. On the other hand, dried fruit generally contains a lot of antioxidants, especially polyphenols. It has been proven that eating dried fruits can prevent heart disease and some types of cancer.

- **NUTS & SEEDS**

Nuts and seeds offer different dietary benefits. They do not only ensure essential nutrients but are also offer a variety of flavors. This "ready to eat" food is a perfect snack with dried fruits and trail mix, essential vegan foods to stockpile for an emergency.

- **RICE & GRAINS**

Rice and grains are versatile and easy to incorporate into your diet. Leftovers reheat wonderfully and can be served at any time of the day, turning simple and inexpensive ingredients into a full-fledged meal. You can also make healthy nut butters such as tahini or peanut butter.

- **BEANS & LEGUMES**

Legumes and beans are highly affordable, and there's no end to the variety of tasty dishes you can cook with them. These humble but powerful foods are packed with vitamins, minerals, protein, and dietary fiber. In addition to being super-healthy and versatile, legumes pair very well with other proteins, vegetables, and grains.

- **HEALTHY FATS**

Don't underestimate the importance of quality fats in cooking. Coconut oil, olive oil, and avocado are always good to have on hand.

- **NON-DAIRY PRODUCTS**

Using a plant-based cheese or milk lends flavor, texture, and nutrition to your meals. You can find fantastic products on the market, and this book has many wonderful recipes for feta, vegan ricotta, and plant-based milk.

- **HERBS, SPICES & CONDIMENTS**

A handful of fresh herbs will add that little something extra to your soups, stews, dips, or casseroles. Condiments such as mustard, ketchup, vegan mayonnaise, and plant-based sauces can be used in salads, casseroles, and spreads. Choosing their distinctive flavors to complement vegetables, grains and legumes will help you to make the most of your vegan dishes. Herbs and spices are naturally plant-based, but play it safe and look for a label that says *Vegan-friendly*.

- **BAKING GOODS & CANNED GOODS**

These vegan essentials include all types of flour, baking powder, baking soda, and yeast. Further, cocoa powder, vegan chocolate, and sweeteners are good to have on hand. As for the healthy vegan sweeteners, opt for fresh or dried fruits, agave syrup, maple syrup, and stevia. When it comes to canned goods, stock your pantry with cooking essentials such as tomato, sauerkraut, pickles, low sodium chickpeas and beans, coconut milk, green chilies, pumpkin puree, tomato sauce, low sodium corn, and artichoke hearts. Thus, if you want to make sure you have nutritious, delicious, and quality meals for you and your family, having a vegan pantry is halfway there.

Why You Ought to Reduce Your Intake of Processed and Animal-Based Foods

You have heard over and over that processed food has adverse effects on your health. You might have also been told repeatedly to stay away from foods with lots of preservatives. However, you may have never heard any genuine or concrete facts about why these foods are unsafe. Consequently, let us properly dissect it to help you properly comprehend why you ought to stay away from these offenders.

- **They have massive habit-forming characteristics**

Humans have a predisposition toward being addicted to some specific foods; however, the reality is that the fault is not wholly ours.

Every one of the unhealthy treats we relish now and then triggers a dopamine release. This creates a pleasurable effect in our brain, but the excitement is usually short-lived. The discharged dopamine gradually causes an attachment, and this is the reason some people consistently go back to eat certain unhealthy foods even when they know they're unhealthy and unnecessary. You can get rid of this by avoiding the temptation completely.

- **They are sugar-laden and heavy in glucose-fructose syrup**

Animal-based and processed foods are laden with refined sugars and glucose-fructose syrup, which has almost no nutritional value. An ever-increasing number of studies are affirming what several people presumed from the start: that genetically modified foods bring about inflammatory bowel disease, which consequently makes it increasingly difficult for the body to assimilate essential nutrients. The disadvantages that result from your body being unable to assimilate essential nutrients from consumed foods rightly cannot be overemphasized.

Processed and animal-based food products contain plenteous amounts of refined carbohydrates. Indeed, your body requires carbohydrates to give it energy to function.

In any case, refining carbs dispenses with the fundamental supplements in the way that refining entire grains disposes of the whole grain part. What remains in the wake of refining is what's considered empty carbs or empty calories. These can negatively affect the metabolic system in your body by sharply increasing your blood sugar and insulin levels.

- **They contain lots of synthetic ingredients**

When your body takes in non-natural ingredients, it regards them as of foreign substance and a health threat. It isn't accustomed to identifying synthetic compounds like sucralose or synthesized sugars. Hence, in defense of your health against this foreign "aggressor," your body does what it's programmed to do to safeguard your health: It sets off an

6

immune reaction to tackle this "enemy" compound, which indirectly weakens your body's general disease alertness, making you susceptible to illnesses. The energy expended by your body in triggering your immune system could be better utilized somewhere else.

- **They contain constituent elements that set off a sensation in your body**

A part of processed and animal-based foods contains compounds like glucose-fructose syrup, monosodium glutamate, and specific food dyes that can trigger some addictions. They teach your body to receive a benefit whenever you consume them. Monosodium glutamate, for example, is added to many store-bought baked foods. This additive slowly conditions your palate to relish and crave the taste.

- **This reward-centric arrangement makes you crave it increasingly, which ends up exposing you to the danger of over-consuming calories**

For animal protein, usually, the expression "subpar" is used to allude to plant proteins since they generally have lower levels of essential amino acids as against animal-sourced protein. Nevertheless, what the vast majority don't know is that large amounts of essential amino acids can prove detrimental to your health. Let me break it down further for you.

- **Animal-sourced protein has no fiber**

In their pursuit to consume animal protein, the vast majority wind up dislodging the plant protein that was previously available in their body. Replacing the plant proteins with its animal variant is harmful because, in contrast to plant protein, animal proteins typically are deficient in fiber, phyto-nutrients, and antioxidant properties. Fiber insufficiency is a regular feature across various regions and societies on the planet. In America, for example, according to the National Academy of Medicine, the typical adult takes in roughly 15 grams of dietary fiber daily rather than the recommended daily quantity of 25 to 30 grams. A deficiency in dietary fiber often leads to a heightened risk of breast and colorectal cancers, in addition to constipation, inflammatory bowel disease, and cardiovascular disease.

- **Animal protein brings about an upsurge in phosphorus levels in the body**

Animal protein has significant levels of phosphorus. Our bodies stabilize these plenteous amounts of phosphorus by producing and discharging a hormone known as fibroblast growth factor 23 (FGF23). Studies have shown that this hormone is dangerous to our veins. FGF23 also causes asymmetrical expansion of heart muscles—a determinant for congestive heart failure and even mortality in some advanced cases.

Having discussed the many problems associated with animal protein, it becomes more apt to replace its "high quality" perception with the tag "highly hazardous." In contrast to caffeine, which has a withdrawal effect if it's discontinued abruptly, you can stop taking processed and animal-based foods right away without any withdrawals. Possibly the only thing that you'll give up is the ease of some meals taking little to no time to prepare.

Health Benefits of the Plant-Based Diet

Plant-based eating is one of the healthiest diets in the world. It should include plenty of fresh products, whole grains, legumes, and healthy fats such as seeds and nuts, which are rich in antioxidants, minerals, vitamins, and dietary fiber.

Scientific research has shown that higher use of plant-based foods is connected to a lower risk of death from conditions such as cardiovascular disease, diabetes, hypertension, and obesity. Vegan eating relies heavily on healthy staples, avoiding animal products. Animal products contain much more fat than plant-based foods; it's not a shocker that studies have shown that meat-eaters have nine times the obesity rate of vegans.

This leads us to the next point, one of the greatest benefits of the vegan diet: weight loss. While many people choose to live a vegan life for ethical reasons, the diet itself can help you achieve your weight loss goals. If you're struggling to shift pounds, you may want to consider trying a plant-based diet. How exactly? As a vegan, you will reduce the number of high-calorie foods such as full-fat dairy products, fatty fish, pork, and other cholesterol-containing foods such as eggs. Try replacing such foods with high-fiber and protein-rich alternatives that will keep you fuller longer. The key is focusing on nutrient-dense, clean and natural foods and avoiding empty calories such as sugar, saturated fats, and highly processed foods. Here are a few tricks that help me maintain my weight on the vegan diet. I eat vegetables as a main course; I consume good fats in moderation (good fats such as olive oil do not make you fat); I exercise regularly and cook at home. Plant foods are an excellent source of many nutrients that boost the body's metabolism in many ways. They are easy to digest thanks to their rich content of antioxidants.

- **Reduced Risk of Heart Diseases**

Processed and animal foods are responsible for much heart disease. A whole foods plant-based diet is better at nourishing the body with essential nutrients while improving the heart's function to produce and transport blood to and from the various body parts.

- **Prevents and Heals Diabetes**

Plant-based foods are excellent at reducing high blood sugar. Many studies comparing a vegetarian and vegan diet to a regular meat-filled diet proved that dieting with more plant foods reduced the risk of diabetes by 50 percent.

- **Improved Cognitive Incline**

Fruits and vegetables are excellent for cleansing and boosting metabolism. They release high numbers of plant compounds and antioxidants that slow or prevent cognitive decline. On a plant-based diet, the brain is boosted with sustainable energy, promoting sharp memory, language, thinking, and judgment abilities.

- **Quick Weight Loss**

A high animal food diet is known to drive weight gain. Switching to a plant-based diet helps the body shed fat walls easily, which quickly drives weight loss.

BREAKFAST

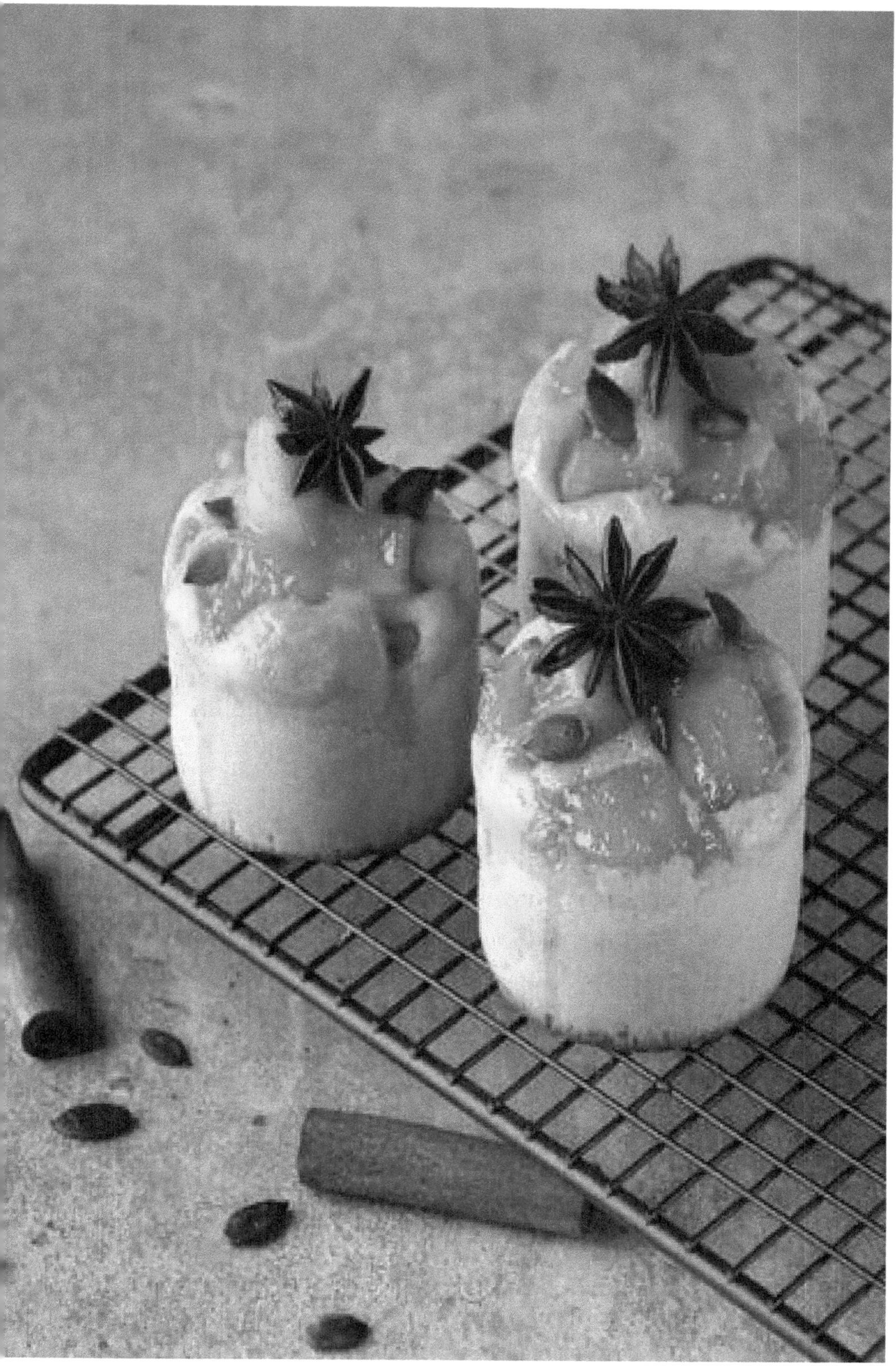

Simple Apple Muffins

6 Servings

Preparation Time: 40 minutes

Ingredients

For the muffin

- 1 Flax seed powder + 3 tbsp water
- 2 tsps Baking powder
- ¼ tsp Salt
- 1 tsp Cinnamon powder
- 1/3 cup melted Plant butter
- 1/3 cup flax Milk
- 1 ½ cups Whole-wheat flour
- ¾ cup Pure date sugar
- 2 Apples, chopped

For topping

- 1/3 cup Whole-wheat flour
- ½ cup cold Plant butter, cubed
- 1 ½ tsps Cinnamon powder
- ½ cup Pure date sugar

Directions

- Preheat oven to 400°F and grease 6 muffin cups with cooking spray.

- In a bowl, mix the flax seed powder with water and allow thickening for 5 minutes to make the vegan "flax egg."

- In a bowl, mix flour, date sugar, baking powder, salt, and cinnamon powder.

- Mix in the butter, vegan "flax egg," flax milk, and fold in the apples. Fill the muffin cups two-thirds way up with the batter.

- In a bowl, mix remaining flour, date sugar, cold butter, and cinnamon powder.

- Sprinkle the mixture on the muffin batter. Bake for 20 minutes.

- Remove the muffins onto a wire rack, allow cooling, and serve.

Almond Yogurt with Berries & Walnuts

6 Servings

Preparation Time: 10 minutes

Ingredients

- 4 cups Almond milk
- 2 tbsps Pure malt syrup
- 2 cups Mixed berries, chopped
- ¼ cup chopped toasted Walnuts
- Dairy-Free Yogurt, cold

Directions

- In a medium bowl, mix the yogurt and malt syrup until well-combined.

- Divide the mixture into 6 breakfast bowls. Top with the berries and walnuts.

- Enjoy immediately.

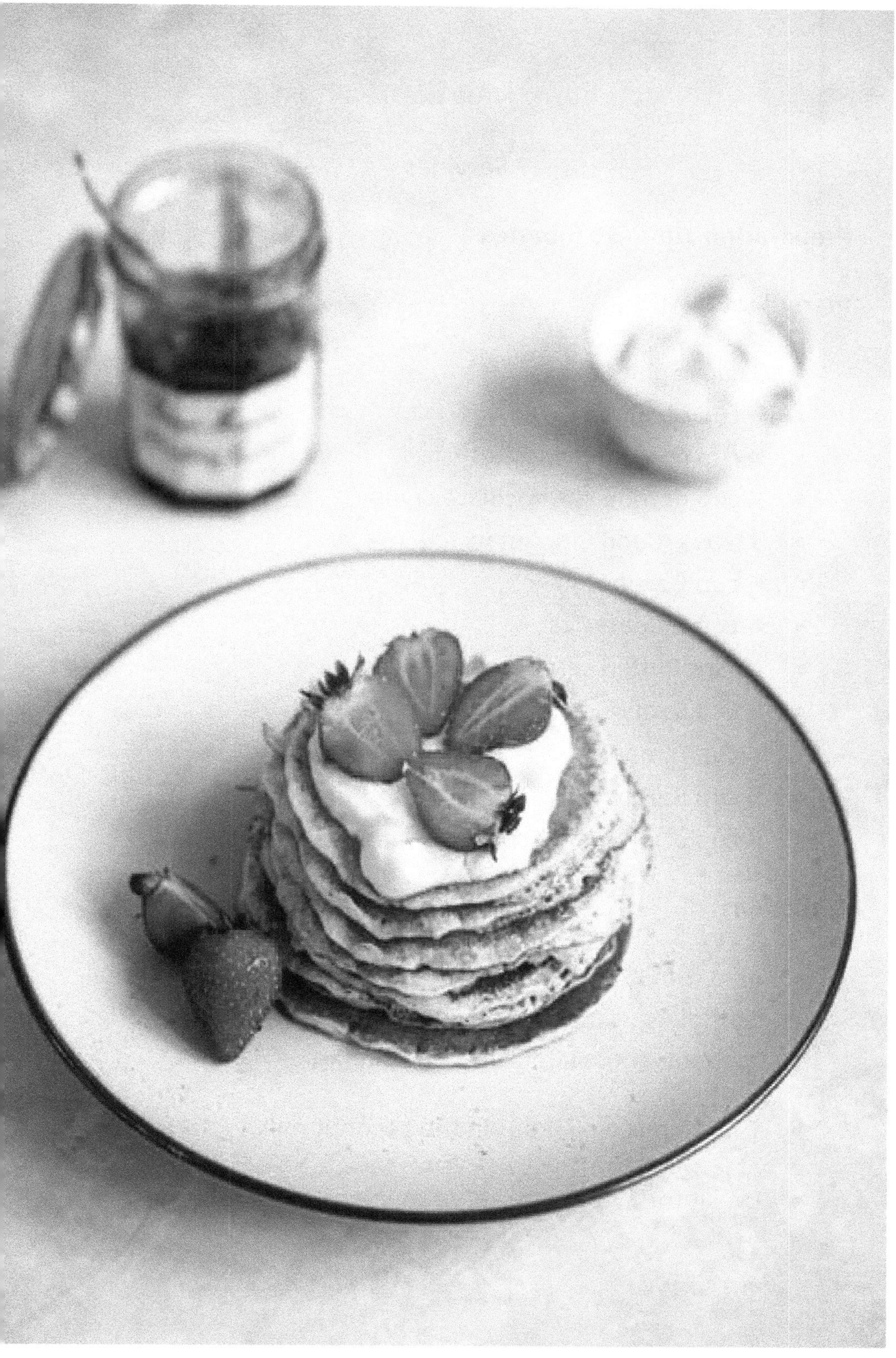

Blueberry Muesli Breakfast

7 Servings

Preparation Time: 10 minutes

Ingredients

- 2 cups Spelt flakes
- ¼ cup chopped Dried figs
- ¼ cup shredded coconut
- ¼ cup non-dairy Chocolate chips
- 3 tsps ground Cinnamon
- ½ cup Coconut milk
- ½ cup Blueberries
- 2 cups Puffed cereal
- ¼ cup Sunflower seeds
- ¼ cup Almonds
- ¼ cup Raisins
- ¼ cup dried Cranberries

Directions

- In a bowl, combine the spelt flakes, puffed cereal, sunflower seeds, almonds, raisins, cranberries, figs, coconut, chocolate chips, and cinnamon.

- Toss to mix well. Pour in the coconut milk.

- Let sit for 1 hour and serve topped with blueberries.

Chocolate-Mango Quinoa Bowl

4 Servings

Preparation Time: 35 minutes

Ingredients

- 1 cup Quinoa
- 3 tbsps unsweetened Cocoa powder
- 2 tbsps Almond butter
- 1 tbsp Hemp seeds
- 1 tbsp Walnuts
- ¼ cup Raspberries
- 1 tsp ground Cinnamon
- 1 cup non-dairy Milk
- 1 large mango, chopped

Directions

- In a pot, mix the quinoa, cinnamon, milk, and 1 cup of water over medium heat.
- Bring to a boil, low heat, and simmer covered for 25-30 minutes.
- In a bowl, mash the mango and mix cocoa powder, almond butter, and hemp seeds.
- In a serving bowl, place cooked quinoa and mango mixture.
- Top with walnuts and raspberries. Serve immediately.

Orange-Carrot Muffins with Cherries

8 Servings

Preparation Time: 45 minutes

Ingredients

- 1 tsp Vegetable oil
- 1 tsp Pure vanilla extract
- ½ tsp ground Cinnamon
- ½ tsp ground Ginger
- ¼ tsp ground Nutmeg
- ¼ tsp Allspice
- ¾ cup Whole-wheat flour
- 1 tsp Baking powder
- ½ tsp Baking soda
- ½ cup Rolled oats
- 2 tbsps Raisins
- 2 tbsps Sunflower seeds
- 2 tbsps Almond butter
- ¼ cup Non-dairy milk
- 1 Orange, peeled
- 1 Carrot, coarsely chopped
- 2 tbsps chopped dried Cherries
- 3 tbsps Molasses
- 2 tbsps ground Flaxseed
- 1 tsp Apple cider vinegar

Directions

- Preheat oven to 350°F. Grease 8 muffin cups with vegetable oil.

- In a blender, add the almond butter, milk, orange, carrot, cherries, molasses, flaxseed, vinegar, vanilla, cinnamon, ginger, nutmeg, and allspice and blend until smooth.

- In a bowl, mix the flour, baking powder, and baking soda. Fold in the wet mixture and gently stir to combine.

- Mix in the oats, raisins, and sunflower seeds.

- Divide the batter between muffin cups. Put in a baking tray and bake for 30 minutes. Serve immediately.

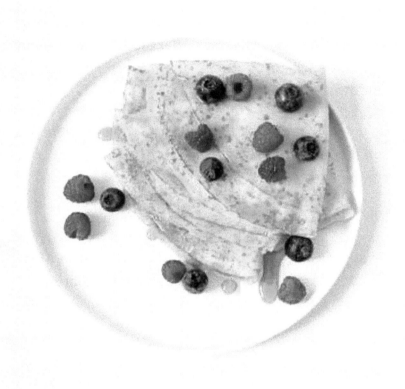

Lemony Quinoa Muffins

7 Servings

Preparation Time: 25 minutes

Ingredients

- 2 tbsps Coconut oil melted, plus more for coating the muffin tin
- 1 tsp Apple cider vinegar
- 2 ½ cups Whole-wheat flour
- 1 ½ cups cooked Quinoa
- 2 tsps Baking soda
- A pinch of salt
- ½ cup Raisins
- ¼ cup ground Flaxseed
- 2 cups unsweetened Lemon curd
- ½ cup Pure date sugar

Directions

- Preheat oven to 400°F.

- In a bowl, mix the flaxseed and ½ cup water.

- Stir in the lemon curd, sugar, coconut oil, and vinegar. Add in the flour, quinoa, baking soda, and salt. Put in the raisins, be careful not too fluffy.

- Divide the batter between greased with coconut oil cups of the tin and bake for 20 minutes until golden and set.

- Allow cooling slightly before removing it from the tin. Serve.

DRINKS

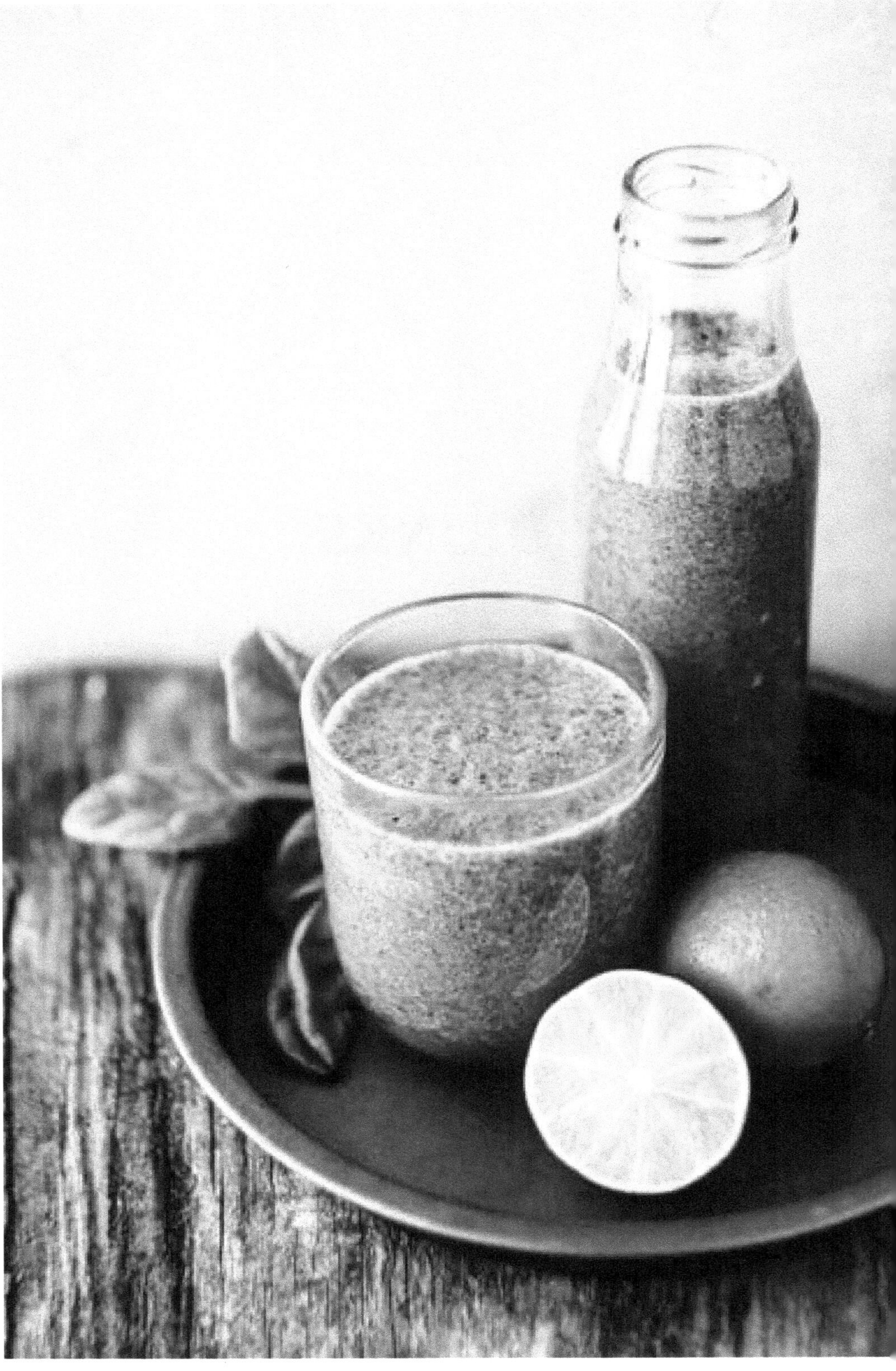

Green Fruity Smoothie

2 Servings

Preparation Time: 15 minutes

Ingredients

- 1 cup of frozen mango, peeled, pitted, and chopped
- 1 large frozen banana, peeled
- 2 cups fresh baby spinach
- 1 scoop unsweetened vegan vanilla protein powder
- ¼ cup pumpkin seeds
- 2 tablespoons hemp hearts
- 1½ cups unsweetened almond milk

Directions

- In a high-speed blender, place all the ingredients and pulse until creamy.
- Pour into two glasses and serve immediately.

Health Boosting Juices

2 Servings

Preparation Time: 15 minutes

Ingredients

For a red juice

- 4 beetroots, quartered
- 2 cups of strawberries
- 2 cups of blueberries
- Ingredients for an orange juice:
- 4 green or red apples, halved
- 10 carrots
- ½ lemon, peeled
- 1" of ginger

For a yellow juice

- 2 green or red apples, quartered
- 4 oranges, peeled and halved
- ½ lemon, peeled
- 1" of ginger

For lime juice

- 6 stalks of celery
- 1 cucumber
- 2 green apples, quartered
- 2 pears, quartered

- Ingredients for a green juice:
- ½ a pineapple, peeled and sliced
- 8 leaves of kale
- 2 fresh bananas, peeled

Directions

- Juice all ingredients in a juicer, chill, and serve.

Thai Iced Tea

4 Servings

Preparation Time: 5 minutes

Ingredients

- 4 cups of water
- 1 can of light coconut milk (14 oz.)
- ¼ cup of maple syrup
- ¼ cup of muscovado sugar
- 1 teaspoon of vanilla extract
- 2 tablespoons of loose-leaf black tea

Directions

- In a large saucepan, over medium heat, bring the water to a boil.
- Turn off the heat and add in the tea, cover and let steep for five minutes.
- Strain the tea into a bowl or jug. Add the maple syrup, muscovado sugar, and vanilla extract. Give it a good whisk to blend all the ingredients.
- Set in the refrigerator to chill. Upon serving, pour ¾ of the tea into each glass, top with coconut milk, and stir.

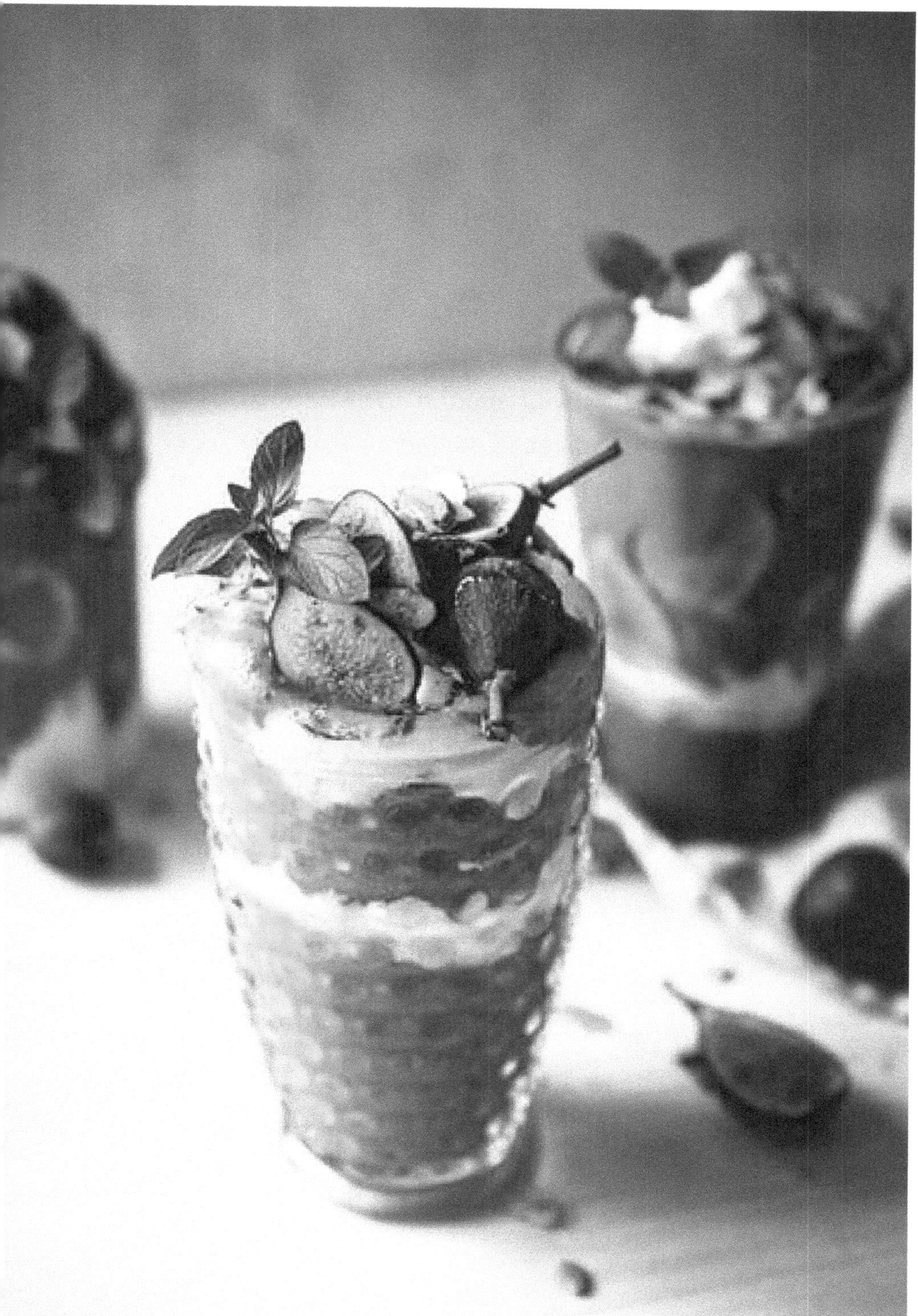

Hot Chocolate

2 Servings

Preparation Time: 5 minutes

Ingredients

- Pinch of brown sugar
- 2 cups of milk, soy or almond, unsweetened
- 2 tablespoons of cocoa powder
- ½ cup of vegan chocolate

Directions

- In a medium saucepan, over medium heat, gently bring the milk to a boil. Whisk in the cocoa powder.
- Remove from the heat; add a pinch of sugar and chocolate. Give it a good stir until smooth, serve, and enjoy.

LUNCH

Black Olive & Chickpea Lunch

6 Servings

Preparation Time: 15 minutes

Ingredients

- 2 tbsps olive oil
- 1 1/3 cups canned chickpeas
- ½ cup pitted black olives
- 1 tbsp chopped fresh oregano
- Salt and black pepper to taste
- 2 cups chopped onion
- 2 garlic cloves, minced
- 2 carrots, cut into thick slices
- 1/3 cup white wine
- 3 cups cherry tomatoes
- 2/3 cup vegetable stock

Directions

- Heat the olive oil in a medium pot and sauté the onion, garlic, and carrots until softened, 5 minutes.

- Mix in the white wine, reduce one-third, and mix in the tomatoes and vegetable stock.

- Cover the lid and cook until the tomatoes break, soften, and the liquid reduces by half.

- Stir in the chickpeas, olives, oregano, and season with salt and pepper. Cook for 3 minutes to warm the chickpeas.

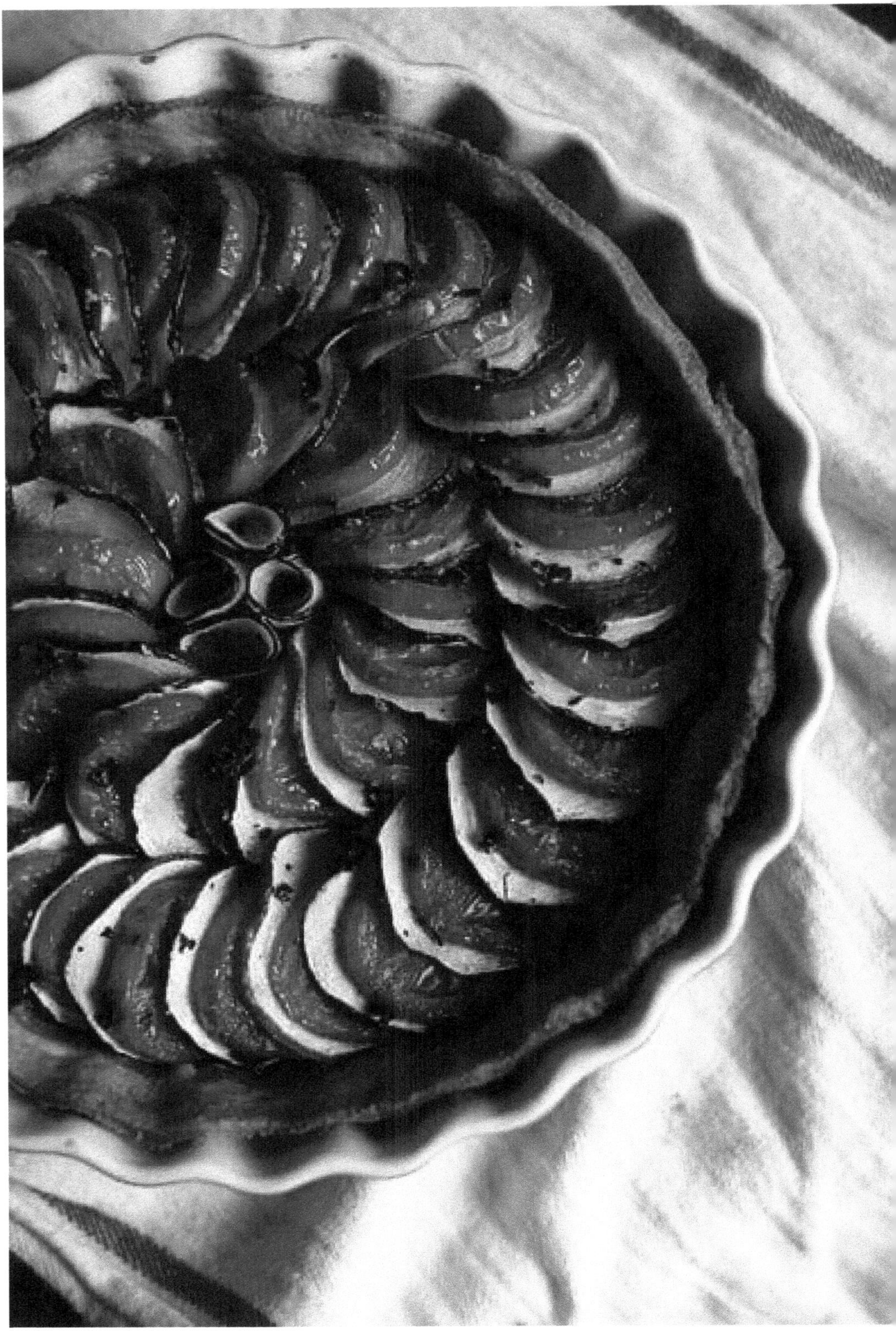

Basil & Tofu Stuffed Portobello Mushrooms

6 Servings

Preparation Time: 25 minutes

Ingredients

- 4 large Portobello mushrooms, stems removed
- ¼ cup crumbled tofu cheese
- 1 tbsp chopped fresh basil
- Garlic salt and black pepper to taste
- ½ tsp olive oil
- 1 small onion, chopped
- 1 cup chopped fresh kale

Directions

- Preheat the oven to 350 F and grease a baking sheet with cooking spray.

- Lightly oil the mushrooms with some cooking spray and season with black pepper and garlic salt.

- Arrange the mushrooms on the baking sheet and bake in the oven until tender, 10 to 15 minutes.

- Heat olive oil in a skillet and sauté onion until tender, 3 minutes. Stir in kale until wilted, 3 minutes. Spoon the mixture into the mushrooms and top with the tofu cheese and basil. Serve.

Kale Pizza with Grilled Zucchini

6 Servings

Preparation Time: 30 minutes

Ingredients

- ¼ cup capers
- ½ cup grated plant Parmesan cheese
- 3 ½ cups whole-wheat flour
- 1 tsp yeast
- 1 tsp salt
- 1 pinch sugar
- 3 tbsps olive oil
- 1 cup marinara sauce
- 2 large zucchinis, sliced
- ½ cup chopped kale
- 1 tsp oregano

Directions

- Preheat the oven the 350 F and lightly grease a pizza pan with cooking spray.

- In a bowl, mix flour, nutritional yeast, salt, sugar, olive oil, and 1 cup of warm water until smooth dough forms.

- Allow rising for an hour or until the dough doubles in size. Spread the dough on the pizza pan and apply marinara sauce and oregano on top.

- Heat a grill pan, season the zucchinis with salt, black pepper, and cook in the pan until slightly charred on both sides.

- Sit the zucchini on the pizza crust and top with kale, capers, and plant-based Parmesan cheese. Bake for 20 minutes. Cool for 5 minutes, slice, and serve.

Amazing Tofu Burgers

6 Servings

Preparation Time: 20 minutes

Ingredients

- 1 tbsp flax seed powder
- ½ tsp garlic powder
- ½ tsp onion powder
- ¼ tsp curry powder
- 3 tbsps whole-grain breadcrumbs
- 4 whole-wheat burger buns, halved
- 2/3 lb crumble tofu
- 1 tbsp quick-cooking oats
- 1 tbsp toasted almond flour

Directions

- In a small bowl, mix the flax seed powder with 3 tbsp water and allow thickening for 5 minutes to make the vegan "flax egg." Set aside.

- In a bowl, mix tofu, oats, almond flour, garlic powder, onion powder, salt, pepper, and curry powder.

- Mold 4 patties out of the mixture and brush both sides with the vegan "flax egg." Pour the breadcrumbs onto a plate and coat the cakes in the crumbs until well covered.

- Heat a pan over medium heat and grease with cooking spray.

- Cook the patties on both sides for 10 minutes. Place each patty between each burger bun and top with the guacamole. Serve immediately.

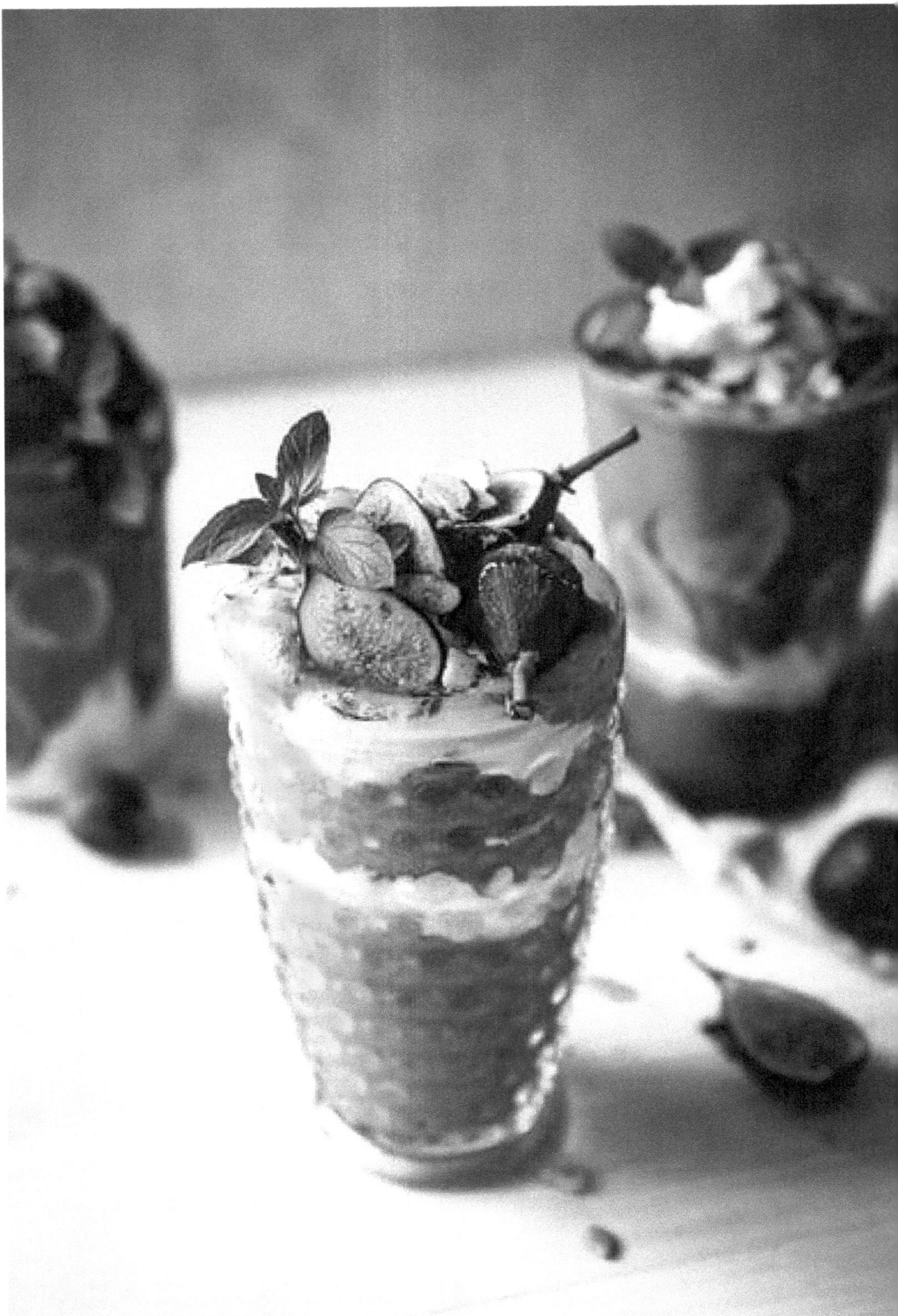

Bean Gyros

6 Servings

Preparation Time: 60 minutes

Ingredients

- 1 (14-oz) can white beans
- 4 tsps olive oil
- 6 whole-grain wraps, warm
- 1 cup hummus
- 1 cup arugula, chopped
- 2 tomatoes, chopped
- 1 cucumber, chopped
- ¼ cup chopped avocado
- 2 scallions, minced
- ¼ cup fresh parsley, chopped
- 2 tbsps Kalamata olives, chopped
- 1 tbsp tahini
- 1 tbsp lemon juice
- ½ tsp ground cumin
- ¼ tsp paprika

Directions

- In a blender, place the white beans, scallions, parsley, and olives. Pulse until finely chopped.

- In a bowl, beat the tahini with lemon juice. Add in cumin, paprika, and salt.

- Transfer into beans mixture and mix well to combine. Shape the mixture into balls; flatten to make 6 patties.

- In a pan over medium heat, warm the oil and cook the patties for 8-10 minutes on both sides; reserve.

- Spread each wrap with hummus and top with patties, tomatoes, cucumber, and avocado. Roll the wraps up to serve.

Saucy Seitan with Sesame Seeds

6 Servings

Preparation Time: 20 minutes

Ingredients

- 4 tsps olive oil
- 1/2 cup soy sauce
- ½ cup + 2 tbsp pure date sugar
- 2 tsps cornstarch
- 1 ½ tbsps olive oil
- 1 lb seitan, cut into 1-inch pieces
- 1 tbsp toasted sesame seeds
- 1 tbsp sliced scallions
- ½ tsp freshly grated ginger
- 3 garlic cloves, minced
- 1/3 tsp red chili flakes
- 1/3 tsp allspice

Directions

- Heat half of the olive oil in a wok and sauté ginger and garlic until fragrant, 30 seconds.

- Mix in red chili flakes, allspice, soy sauce, and date sugar. Allow the sugar to melt and set aside.

- In a small bowl, mix cornstarch and 2 tbsp of water. Stir the cornstarch mixture into the sauce and allow thickening for 1 minute.

- Heat the remaining olive oil in a medium skillet over medium heat and fry the seitan on both sides until crispy, 10 minutes.

- Mix the seitan into the sauce and warm over low heat. Dish the food, garnish with sesame seeds and scallions. Serve warm.

Broccoli Stuffed Cremini Mushrooms

6 Servings

Preparation Time: 35 minutes

Ingredients

- ½ head broccoli, cut into florets
- 1 bell pepper, chopped
- 1 tsp Cajun seasoning mix
- Salt and black pepper, to taste
- ¼ cup plant-based mozzarella
- 1 lb cremini mushroom caps
- 2 tbsps olive oil
- 1 onion, finely chopped
- 1 tsp garlic, minced

Directions

- Preheat oven to 360 F.

- Bake mushroom caps in a greased baking dish for 10-12 minutes.

- In a blende, place broccoli and pulse until it becomes like small rice-like granules. In a heavy-bottomed skillet, warm olive oil; stir in bell pepper, garlic, and onion and sauté until fragrant.

- Place in pepper, salt, and Cajun seasoning mix. Fold in broccoli rice. Divide the filling mixture among mushroom caps.

- Top with plant-based mozzarella cheese and bake for 17 more minutes. Serve warm.

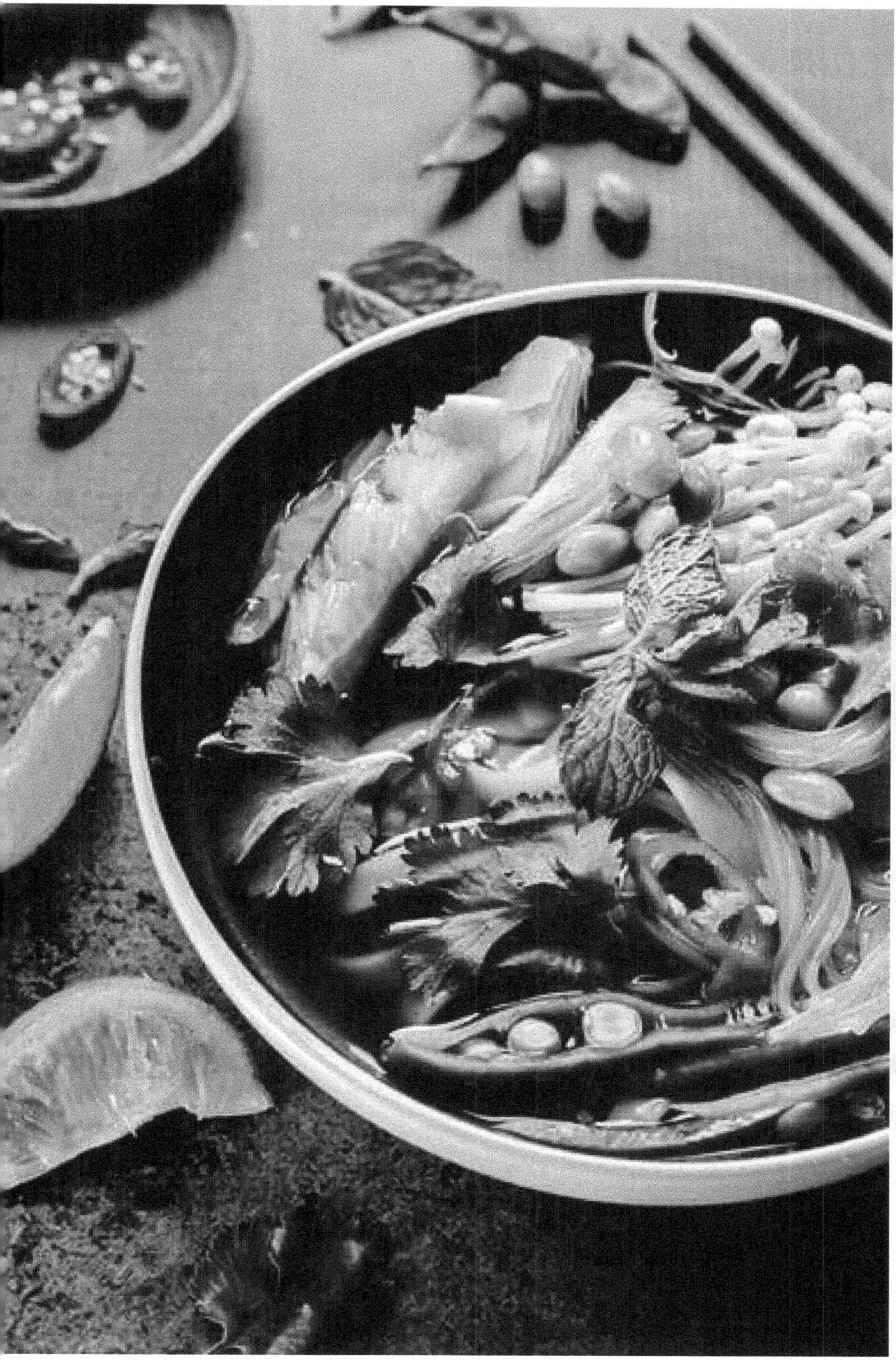

Tempeh & Vegetable Stir-Fry

6 Servings

Preparation Time: 30 minutes

Ingredients

- 1 can (28 oz) whole plum tomatoes
- 1 tbsp pure date sugar
- 1 tsp dried mixed herbs
- 1 small head cabbage, thinly sliced
- 1 green bell pepper, cut into strips
- 1 lb crumbled tempeh
- 1 large yellow onion, chopped
- 1 can (8 oz) tomato sauce
- 2 tbsps plain vinegar

Directions

- Drain the tomatoes and reserve their liquid. Chop the tomatoes and set them aside.

- Add the tempeh to a large skillet and cook until brown, 10 minutes.

- Mix in the onion, tomato sauce, vinegar, date sugar, mixed herbs, and chopped tomatoes.

- Close the lid and cook until the liquid reduces, 10 minutes. Stir in the cabbage and bell pepper; cook until softened, 5 minutes. Serve.

SNACKS & SIDES

Grilled Vegetables with Romesco Dip

8 Servings

Preparation time: 35 minutes

Ingredients

- 2 (12-oz) jar roasted peppers, drained
- 1 cup toasted almonds
- 2 garlic cloves, minced
- 2 tbsps red wine vinegar
- 2 tsps crushed red chili flakes
- 4 slices toasted bread, chopped
- 1 tsp sweet paprika
- 2 tbsps tomato paste
- 1 cup olive oil + 2 tbsp for brushing
- Salt and black pepper to taste
- 2 green bell peppers, julienned
- 2 yellow bell peppers, julienned
- 2 bunch of asparagus, trimmed

Directions

- In a food processor, place roasted peppers, almonds, garlic, vinegar, toasted bread, paprika, and tomato paste;

- pulse, pouring slowly ½ cup of olive oil until the desired consistency is reached.

- Season with salt and black pepper and set aside.

- Heat a grill pan over medium heat.

- Toss the vegetables in the remaining olive oil, season with salt and pepper, and cook in the pan for 3-5 minutes per side.

- Serve with the dip.

Cacao Nut Bites

8 Servings

Preparation time: 5 minutes

Ingredients

- 7 oz dairy-free dark chocolate
- 1 cup mixed nuts
- 4 tbsps roasted coconut chips
- 2 tbsps sunflower seeds
- Sea salt

Directions

- Pour the chocolate into a safe microwave bowl and melt in the microwave for 1 to 2 minutes.

- Into 10 small cupcake liners (2-inches in diameters), share the chocolate.

- Drop in the nuts, coconut chips, sunflower seeds, and sprinkle with some salt. Chill in the refrigerator until firm.

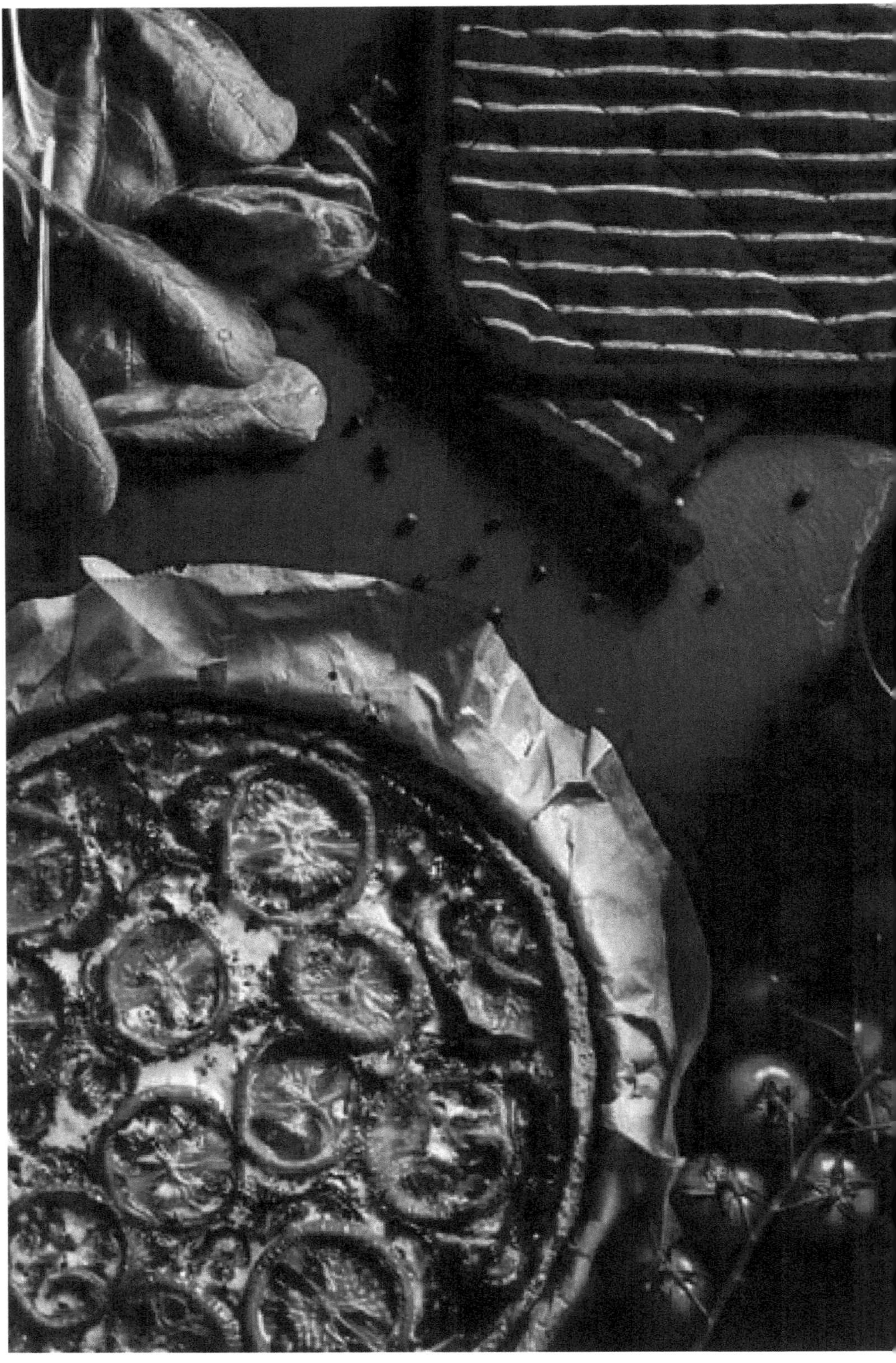

Garbanzo Quesadillas with Salsa

8 Servings

Preparation time: 15 minutes

Ingredients

- 2 (15.5-oz) can garbanzo beans, mashed
- 4 tbsps canola oil
- 2 tsps chili powder
- 16 whole-wheat flour tortilla wraps
- 2 cups tomato salsa
- 1 cup minced red onion

Directions

- Warm the canola oil in a pot over medium heat.

- Place in mashed garbanzo and chili powder, cook for 5 minutes, stirring often. Set aside.

- Heat a pan over medium heat. Put one tortilla in the pan and top with ¼ each of the garbanzo spread, tomato salsa, and onion.

- Cover with other tortilla and cook for 2 minutes, flip the quesadilla and cook for another 2 minutes until crispy.

- Repeat the process with the remaining tortillas. Slice and serve.

Tarragon Potato Chips

8 Servings

Preparation time: 40 minutes

Ingredients

- 2 lbs potato, peeled and sliced
- 2 tsps smoked paprika
- 1 tsp garlic powder
- 2 tbsps tarragon
- ½ tsp onion powder
- ½ tsp chili powder
- ¼ tsp ground mustard
- 2 tsps canola oil
- ¼ tsp liquid smoke

Directions

- Preheat oven to 390 F.

- Combine the paprika, garlic powder, tarragon, onion powder, chili powder, salt, and mustard in a bowl.

- Mix the potatoes, canola oil, liquid smoke, and tarragon mixture in another bowl; toss to coat.

- Spread the potatoes on a lined with parchment paper baking tray and bake for 30 minutes, flipping once halfway through cooking until golden. Serve.

Tamari Lentil Dip

4 Servings

Preparation time: 10 minutes

Ingredients

- 2 (14-oz) can lentils, drained
- Zest and juice of 2 lime
- 2 tbsps tamari sauce
- ½ cup fresh cilantro, chopped
- 2 tsps ground cumin
- 2 tsps cayenne pepper

Directions

- In a blender, put the lentils, lime zest, lime juice, tamari sauce, and ¼ cup of water.

- Pulse until smooth. Transfer to a bowl and stir in cilantro, cumin and cayenne pepper. Serve.

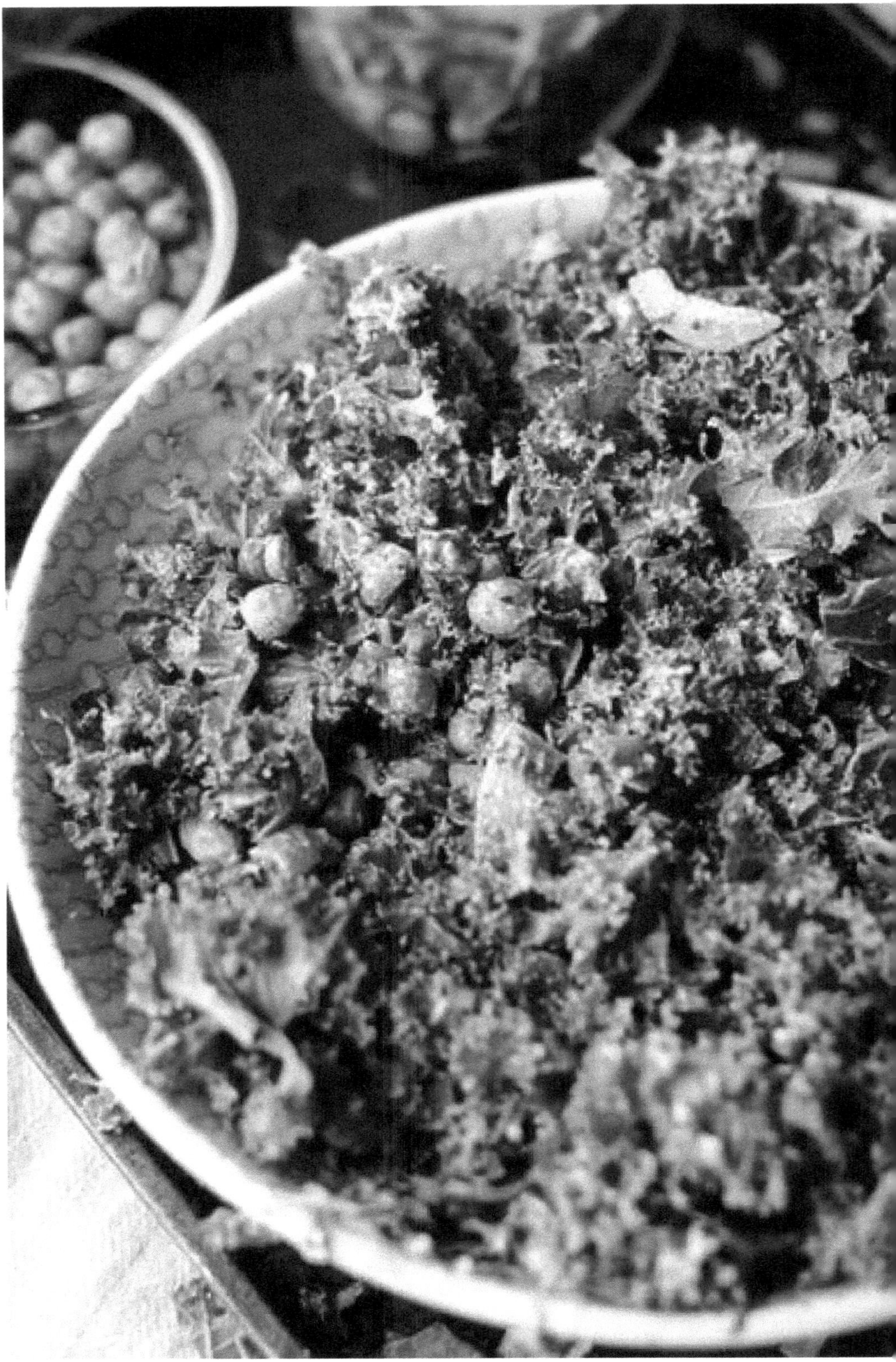

Chili Roasted Hazelnuts

8 Servings

Preparation time: 20 minutes

Ingredients

- 1 lb raw hazelnuts
- 3 tbsps tamari sauce
- 2 tbsps extra-virgin olive oil
- 1 tbsp nutritional yeast
- 2 tsps chili powder

Directions

- Preheat oven to 390 F.

- Combine the hazelnuts, tamari, and oil in a bowl.

- Toss to coat. Spread the mixture on a parchment-lined baking pan and roast for 10-15 minutes until browned.

- Let cool for e few minutes. Sprinkle with yeast and chili powder.

Balsamic Roasted Red Pepper & Pecan Crostini

16 Servings

Preparation time: 15 minutes

Ingredients

- 2 jarred roasted red peppers
- 1 cup unsalted pecans
- ¼ cup water
- 1 tbsp soy sauce
- 2 tbsps chopped green onions
- ¼ cup nutritional yeast
- 2 tbsps balsamic vinegar
- 2 tbsps olive oil

Directions

- Cut 1 red pepper and set aside.

- Slice the remaining pepper into strips, reserve for garnish.

- Pulse the pecans in a food processor until a fine powder forms.

- Pour in water, chopped red pepper, and soy sauce.

- Pulse until smooth. Put in green onions, yeast, vinegar, and oil.

- Blend until well mixed.

- Spread mixture onto toasted bread slices topped with pepper strips.

Bell Peppers Stuffed with Spinach & Tofu

4 Servings

Preparation time: 35 minutes

Ingredients

- 2 tbsps olive oil

- 1 onion, chopped
- 2 garlic cloves, minced
- 1 (14-oz) block tofu, crumbled
- 1 (5-oz) package baby spinach
- 2 tsps Italian seasoning
- Salt and black pepper to taste
- 4 large bell peppers, top removed

Directions

- Preheat oven to 450 F.

- Heat the oil in a skillet over medium heat.

- Place onion and garlic and cook for 3 minutes.

- Put in tofu and spinach and cook for 3 minutes until the spinach wilts.

- Stir in Italian seasoning, salt, and pepper.

- Fill the bell peppers with the spinach mixture and arrange them on a greased baking sheet.

- Bake in the oven for 25 minutes.

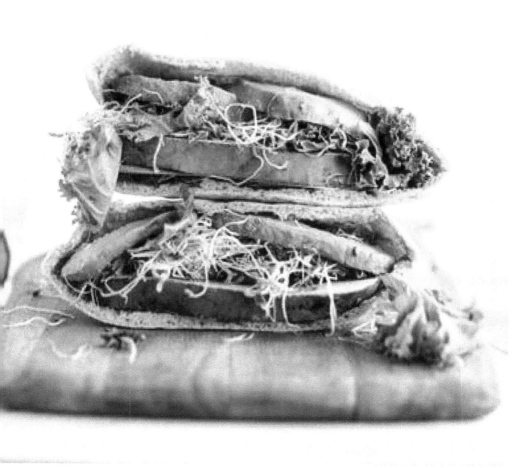

Kale & Hummus Pinwheels

8 Servings

Preparation time: 10 minutes

Ingredients

- 6 whole-grain flour tortillas
- 2 cups kale, chopped
- 3 cups hummus
- 3 cups shredded carrots

Directions

- Spread hummus over tortillas and top with kale and carrots.

- Fold the edges over the filling and roll up to make burritos.

- Cut into pinwheels and serve.

SOUPS & SALADS

Italian Bean Soup

8 Servings

Preparation Time: 1 hour 25 minutes

Ingredients

- 3 tbsps Olive oil
- 6 cups Vegetable broth
- 1 (14.5-oz) can diced Tomatoes
- 2 Bay leaves
- Salt and Black pepper to taste
- 2 (15.5-oz) cans White beans
- ¼ cup chopped Basil
- 2 Celery stalks, chopped
- 2 Carrots, chopped
- 3 Shallots, chopped
- 3 Garlic cloves, minced
- ½ cup Brown rice

Directions

- Warm the oil in a pot over medium heat.

- Add the celery, carrots, shallots, and garlic and cook for 5 minutes.

- Add in brown rice, broth, tomatoes, bay leaves, salt, and pepper.

- Bring to a boil, then lower the heat and simmer uncovered for 20 minutes.

- Stir in beans and basil and cook for 5 minutes.

- Discard bay leaves and spoon into bowls. Sprinkle with basil and serve.

Brussels Sprouts & Tofu Soup

6 Servings

Preparation Time: 40 minutes

Ingredients

- 7 oz firm Tofu, cubed
- ½-inch piece fresh Ginger, minced
- Salt to taste
- 2 tbsps Apple cider vinegar
- 2 tbsps Soy sauce
- 1 tsp Pure date sugar
- ¼ tsp Red pepper flakes
- 1 Scallion, chopped
- 2 tsps Olive oil
- 1 cup sliced Mushrooms
- 1 cup shredded Brussels sprouts
- 1 Garlic clove, minced

Directions

- Warm the oil in a pan over medium heat.

- Add the mushrooms, Brussels sprouts, garlic, ginger, and salt. Sauté for 7-8 minutes until the veggies are soft.

- Pour in 4 cups of water, vinegar, soy sauce, sugar, pepper flakes, and tofu.

- Bring to a boil, then lower the heat and simmer for 5-10 minutes.

- Top with scallions and serve.

Rosemary White Bean Soup

6 Servings

Preparation Time: 30 minutes

Ingredients

- 2 tsps Olive oil
- 1 tbsp Rosemary, chopped
- 2 tbsps Apple cider vinegar
- 1 cup Dried white beans
- ¼ tsp Salt
- 2 tbsps Nutritional yeast
- 1 Carrot, chopped
- 1 Onion, chopped
- 2 Garlic cloves, minced

Directions

- Warm the oil in a pot over medium heat. Place carrots, onion, and garlic and cook for 5 minutes.

- Pour in vinegar to deglaze the pot.

- Stir in 5 cups water and beans and bring to a boil. Lower the heat and simmer for 45 minutes until the beans are soft.

- Add in salt and nutritional yeast and stir. Serve topped with chopped rosemary.

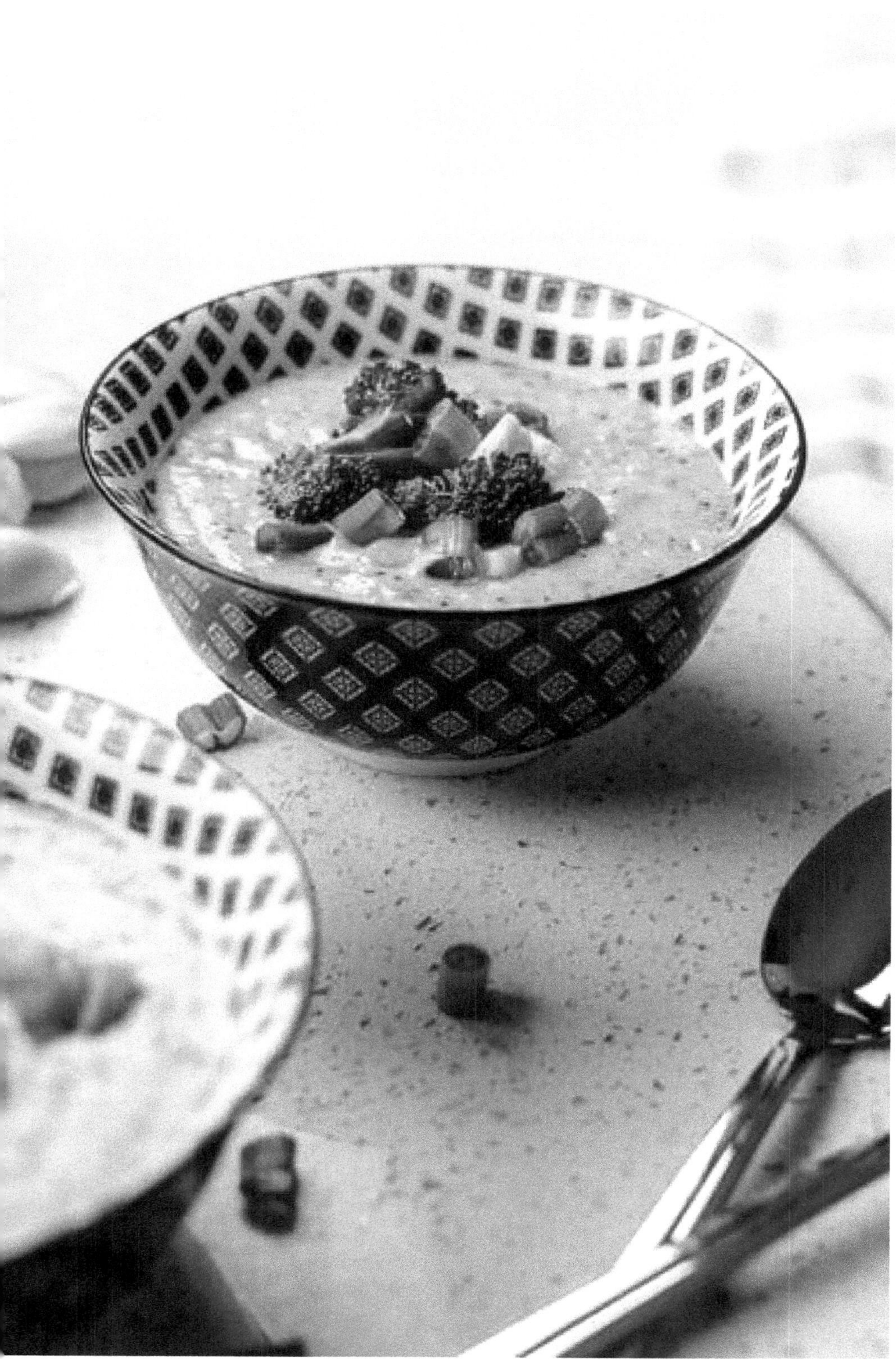

Mushroom & Tofu Soup

6 Servings

Preparation Time: 20 minutes

Ingredients

- 4 cups water
- ¼ cup chopped Green onions
- 3 tbsps Tahini
- 6 oz extra-firm Tofu, diced
- 2 tbsps Soy sauce
- 4 white Mushrooms, sliced

Directions

- Add the water and soy sauce into a pot and bring to a boil.

- Add in mushrooms and green onions. Lower the heat and simmer for 10 minutes.

- In a bowl, combine ½ cup of hot soup with tahini.

- Pour the mixture into the pot and simmer 2 minutes more, but not boil. Stir in tofu.

- Serve warm.

Seitan & Spinach Salad a la Puttanesca

6 Servings

Preparation Time: 11 minutes

Ingredients

- 4 tbsps Olive oil
- 2 tbsps Capers
- 3 cups Baby spinach, cut into strips
- 1 ½ cups Cherry tomatoes, halved
- 2 tbsps Balsamic vinegar
- 2 tbsps Torn fresh basil leaves
- 2 tbsps minced fresh Parsley
- 1 cup Pomegranate seeds
- 8 oz Seitan, cut into strips
- 2 Garlic cloves, minced
- ½ cup Kalamata olives, halved
- ½ cup Green olives, halved

Directions

- Heat half of the olive oil in a pan over medium heat.

- Place the seitan and brown for 5 minutes on all sides.

- Add in garlic and cook for 30 seconds. Remove to a bowl and let cool.

- Stir in olives, capers, spinach, and tomatoes. Set aside.

- In another bowl, whisk the remaining oil, vinegar, salt, and pepper until well mixed.

- Pour this dressing over the seitan salad and toss to coat.

- Top with basil, parsley, and pomegranate seeds. Serve.

Tomato & Avocado Lettuce Salad

6 Servings

Preparation Time: 15 minutes

Ingredients

- 1 Garlic clove, chopped1/3 cup olive oil
- 1 head Iceberg lettuce, shredded
- 12 Ripe grape tomatoes, halved
- ½ cup frozen Peas, thawed
- 8 Black olives, pitted
- 1 Avocado, sliced
- 1 Red onion, sliced
- ½ tsp Dried basil
- Salt and Black pepper to taste
- ¼ tsp pure Date sugar
- 3 tbsps white Wine vinegar

Directions

- In a blender, place the garlic, onion, oil, basil, salt, pepper, sugar, and vinegar.

- Blend until smooth. Set aside. Place the lettuce, tomatoes, peas, and olives on a nice serving plate.

- Top with avocado slices and drizzle the previously prepared dressing all over. Serve.

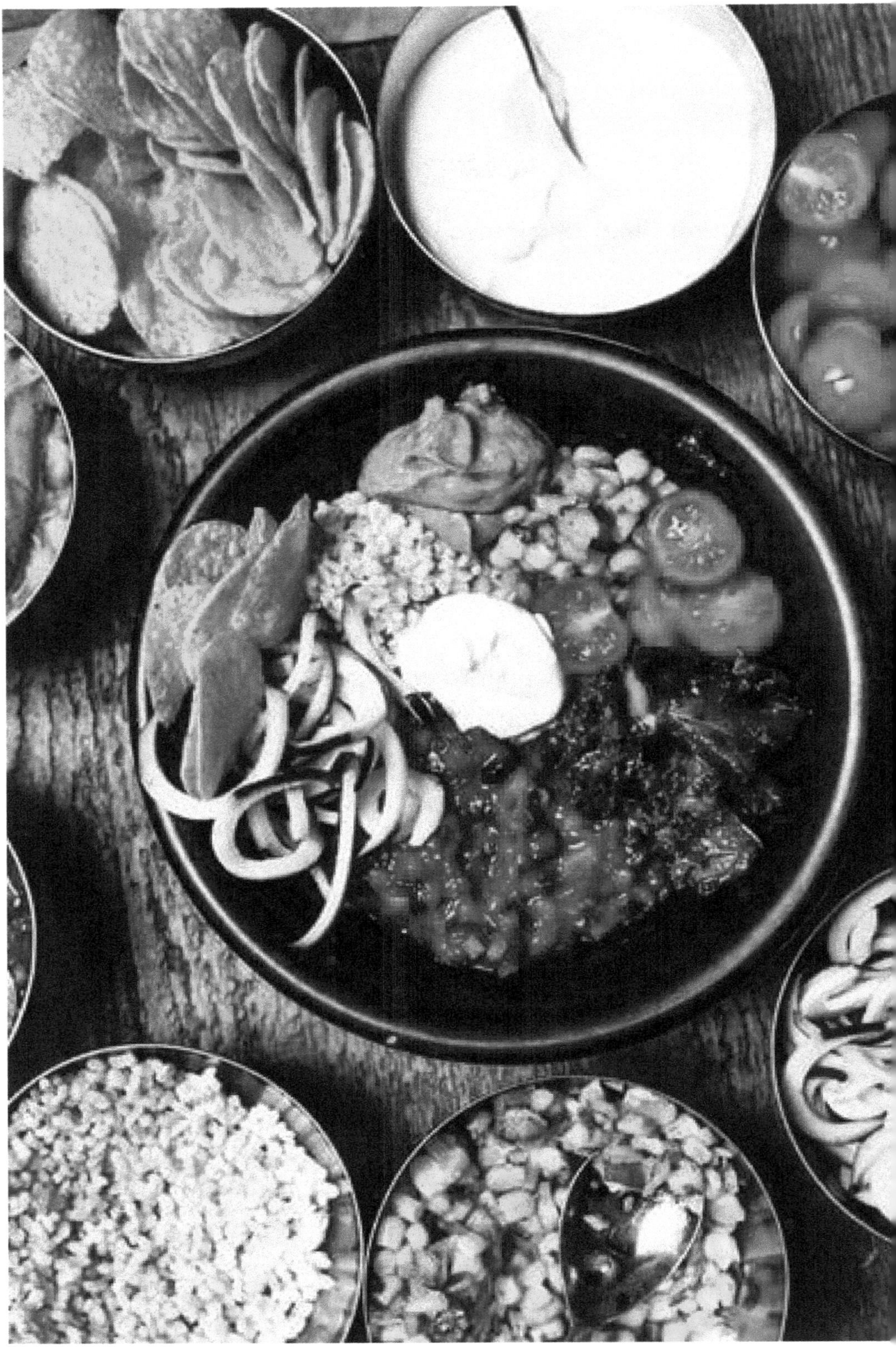

Fried Broccoli Salad with Tempeh & Cranberries

6 Servings

Preparation Time: 15 minutes

Ingredients

- 3 oz Plant butter
- 1 lb Broccoli florets
- Salt and Black pepper to taste
- 2 oz Almonds
- ½ cup frozen Cranberries
- ¾ lb Tempeh slices, cubed

Directions

- In a skillet, melt the plant butter over medium heat until no longer foaming, and fry the tempeh cubes until brown on all sides.

- Add the broccoli and stir-fry for 6 minutes. Season with salt and pepper.

- Turn the heat off. Stir in the almonds and cranberries to warm through.

- Share salad into bowls and serve.

Balsamic Lentil Salad

6 Servings

Preparation Time: 40 minutes

Ingredients

- 2 tsps Olive oil
- 1 cup Lentils
- 1 tbsp dried Basil
- 1 tbsp dried Oregano
- 1 tbsp Balsamic vinegar
- 2 cups water
- Sea salt to taste
- 2 cups chopped Swiss chard
- 2 cups Torn curly endive
- 1 red Onion, diced
- 1 Garlic clove, minced
- 1 Carrot, diced

Directions

- In a bowl, mix the balsamic vinegar, olive oil, and salt. Set aside.

- Warm 1 tsp of oil in a pot over medium heat.

- Place the onion and carrot and cook for 5 minutes.

- Mix in lentils, basil, oregano, balsamic vinegar, and water and bring to a boil.

- Lower the heat and simmer for 20 minutes.

- Mix in two-thirds of the dressing.

- Add in the Swiss chard and cook for 5 minutes on low. Let cool. Coat the endive with the remaining dressing.

- Transfer to a plate and top with lentil mixture to serve.

DINNER

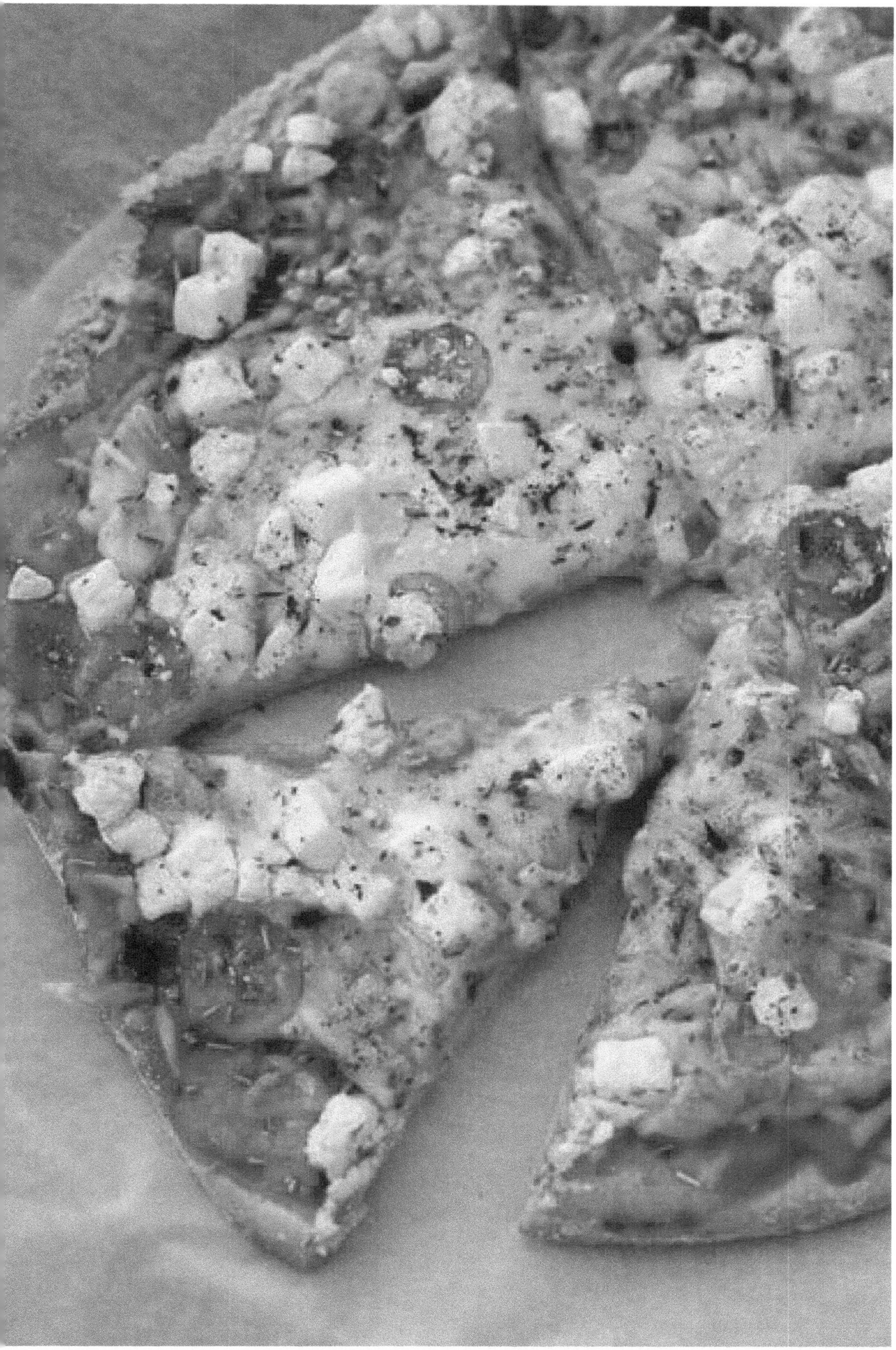

Basil Beet Pasta

6 Serving

Preparation Time: 20 minutes

Ingredients

- 1 tsp Olive oil
- ½ tsp dried basil
- ½ tsp dried oregano
- ½ tsp red Pepper flakes
- 1 Garlic clove, minced
- 4 medium Beets, spiralizer

Directions

- Add oil in a pan, heat it on medium heat.

- Add garlic, beets, basil, oregano, pepper flakes, salt, and pepper.

- Cook for 15 minutes and serve.

Tofu Eggplant Pizza

6 Servings

Preparation Time: 45 minutes

Ingredients

- 2 Eggplants, sliced lengthwise
- 1/3 cup melted Plant butter
- ¼ cup chopped fresh Oregano
- 2 Garlic cloves, minced
- 1 Red Onion
- 12 Oz Crumbled Tofu
- 7 oz Tomato sauce
- ½ tsp Cinnamon powder
- 1 cup grated Plant-based Parmesan

Directions

- Preheat oven to 400 F and line a baking sheet with parchment paper.

- Brush eggplants with some plant butter and transfer it to the baking sheet and bake until lightly browned for about 20 minutes.

- Heat the remaining butter in a skillet and sauté the garlic and onion until fragrant and soft, about 3 minutes.

- Stir in the tofu and cook for 3 minutes and add the tomato sauce and season with salt and black pepper, then simmer for 10 minutes.

- Remove the eggplant from the oven and spread the tofu sauce on top. Sprinkle with plant-based Parmesan cheese and oregano.

- Bake further for 10 minutes or until the cheese has melted. Serve.

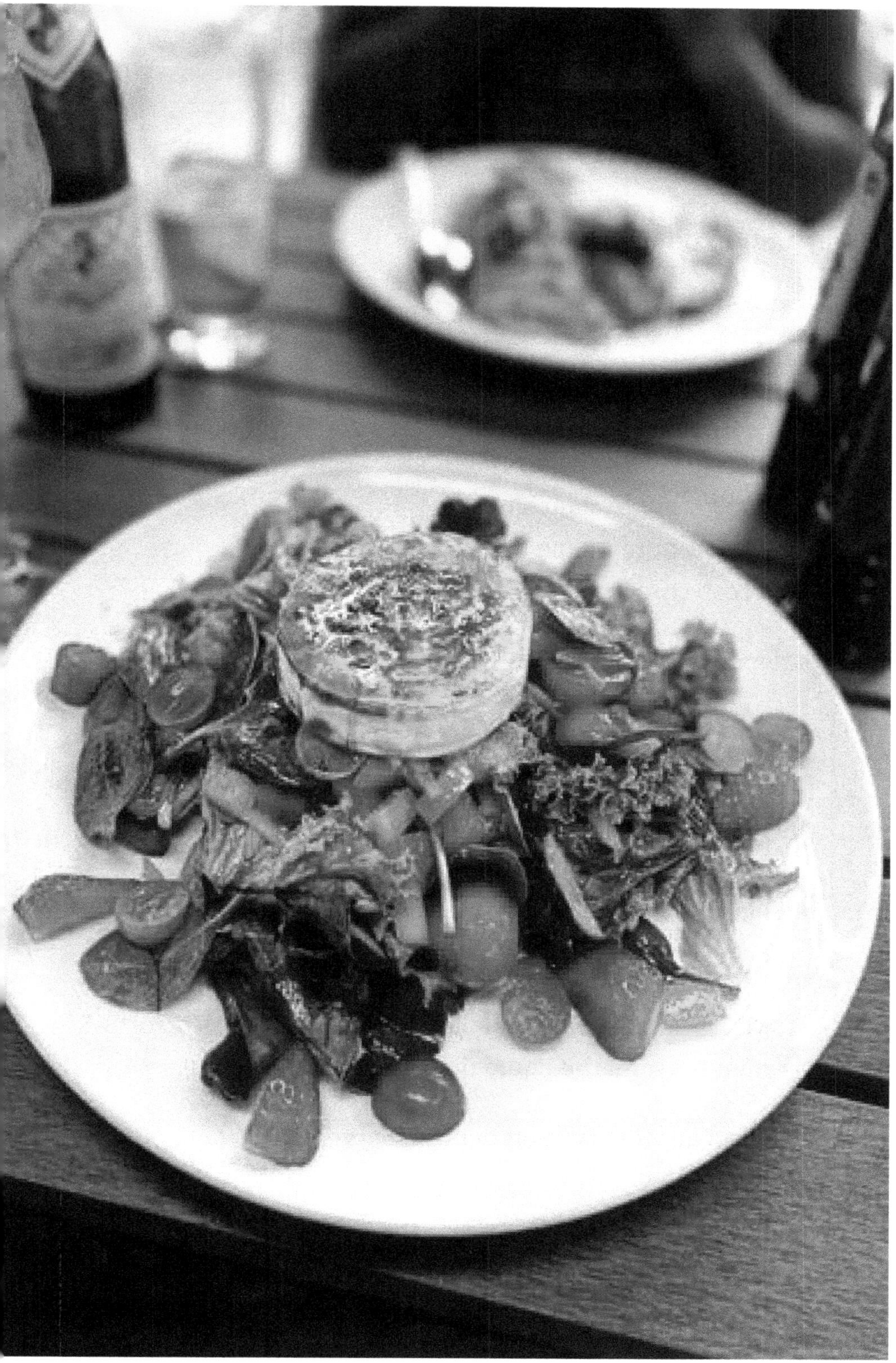

Maple Green Cabbage Hash

8 Servings

Preparation time: 25 minutes

Ingredients

- 6 tbsps olive oil
- 4 shallots, thinly sliced
- 3 lbs green cabbage, shredded
- 6 tbsps apple cider vinegar
- 2 tbsps pure maple syrup
- 1 tbsp sriracha sauce

Directions

- Heat the oil in a skillet over medium temperature.

- Put in shallots and shredded cabbage and heat it for 10 minutes until it becomes tender.

- Put in some vinegar and scrape any bits from the bottom.

- Mix in maple syrup and sriracha sauce. Heat it for 3-5 minutes until the liquid disappears.

- Sprinkle with salt and pepper. Serve right away.

Raisin & Pine Nut Zucchini Rolls

8 Servings

Preparation time: 50 minutes

Ingredients

- 8 zucchinis, sliced lengthwise
- Salt and black pepper to taste
- 4 tbsps olive oil
- 2 garlic cloves, minced
- 8 green onions, chopped
- 1/2 cup ground pine nuts
- 4 tbsps chopped sun-dried tomatoes
- 6 tbsps golden raisins
- 6 tbsps plant-based Parmesan
- 2 tbsps minced fresh parsley
- 4 cups marinara sauce

Directions

- Heat oven to 360 F.

- place the zucchini slices on a greased baking sheet.

- Season with salt and pepper and bake for 15 minutes. Set aside.

- Heat the oil in a skillet over medium temperature.

- Place in garlic, green onions, and pine nuts and heat it for 1 minute.

- Stir in tomatoes, raisins, Parmesan cheese, parsley, salt, and pepper.

- Spread the mixture onto the zucchini slices. Roll up and transfer to the baking dish.

- Top with marinara sauce.

- Cover with foil and bake for 30 minutes. Serve hot.

Almond & Chickpea Patties

12 Servings

Preparation time: 50 minutes

Ingredients

- 2 roasted red bell peppers, chopped
- 2 (19-oz) can chickpeas
- 2 cups ground almonds
- 4 tsps Dijon mustard
- 4 tsps date syrup
- 2 garlic cloves, pressed
- Juice of 1 lemon
- 2 cups kale, chopped
- 2 ½ cups rolled oats

Directions

- Preheat oven to 360 F.

- Line with parchment paper a baking sheet.

- In a blender, put the chickpeas, almonds, bell pepper, mustard, date syrup, garlic, lemon juice, and kale.

- Stir until ingredients are finely chopped but not over blended.

- Add in the oats.

- Shake until everything is well combined.

- Shape the mixture into 12 patties and arrange them on the baking sheet.

- Bake them for 30 minutes until light brown. Serve.

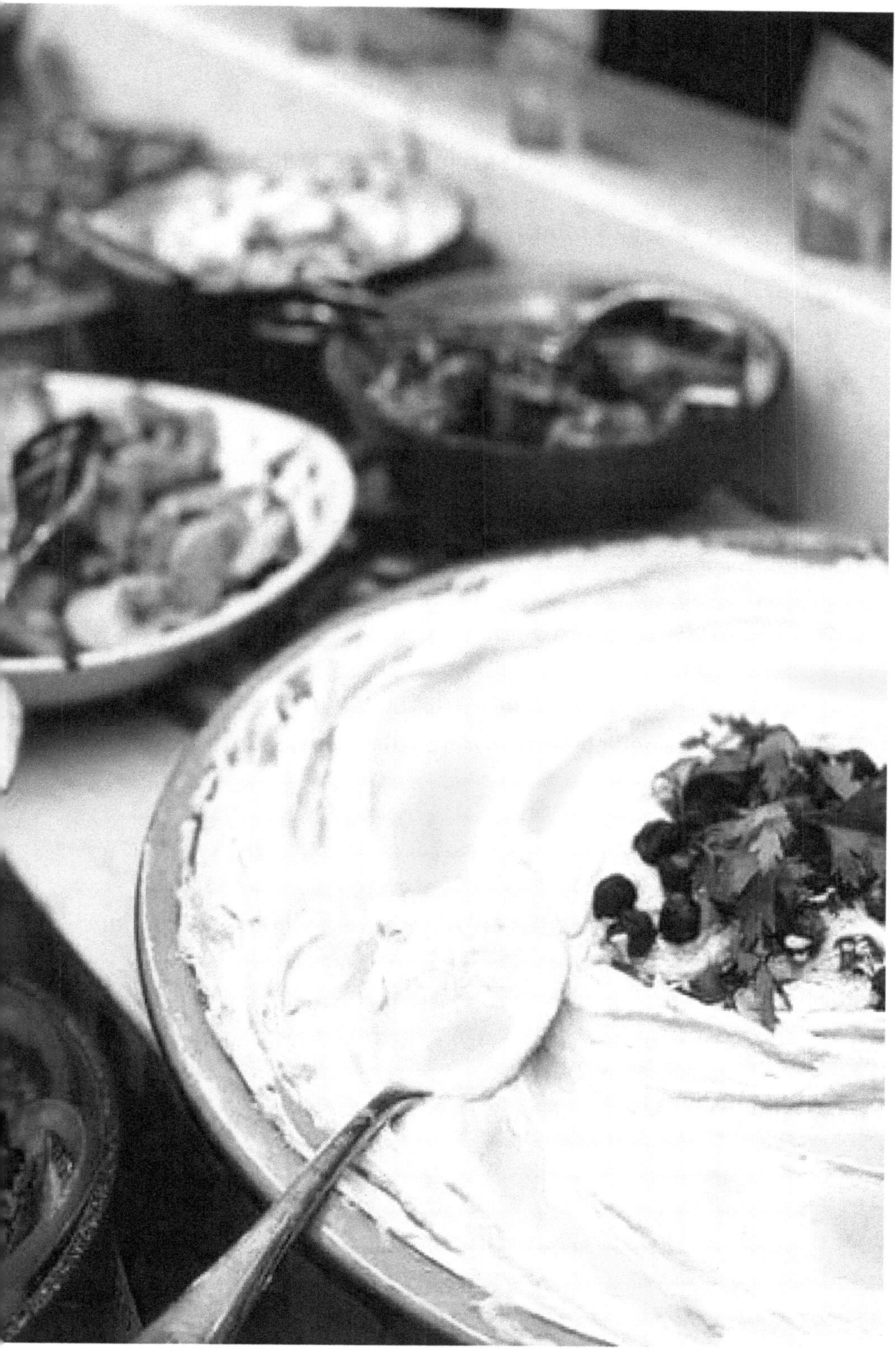

Korean-Style Buckwheat

8 Servings

Preparation time: 25 minutes

Ingredients

- 4 cups water
- 2 cups buckwheat groats, rinsed
- 1/2 cup unseasoned rice vinegar
- ½ cup Mirin wine

Directions

- Heat the water in a pot.

- Put in the buckwheat groats, lower the temperature, and simmer covered for 15-20 minutes until the liquid disappears.

- Let cool for a few minutes.

- Using a fork, fluff the groats and stir in vinegar and Mirin wine. Serve.

Peanut Quinoa & Chickpea Pilaf

8 Servings

Preparation time: 30 minutes

Ingredients

- 2 tbsps olive oil

- 2 medium red onions, minced
- 3 cups quinoa, rinsed
- 6 cups vegetable broth
- 4 (15.5-oz) cans chickpeas
- 1/2 tsp ground cayenne
- 2 tbsps minced fresh chives
- 2 tangerines, chopped
- 1 cup peanuts

Directions

- Heat the oil in a skillet over medium temperature.

- Put the onion and heat for 3 minutes until softened.

- Add in quinoa and broth.

- Heat till boil, then lower the heat and sprinkle with salt.

- Simmer for 20 minutes.

- Put in chickpeas, cayenne pepper, chives, tangerine, and peanuts. Serve warm.

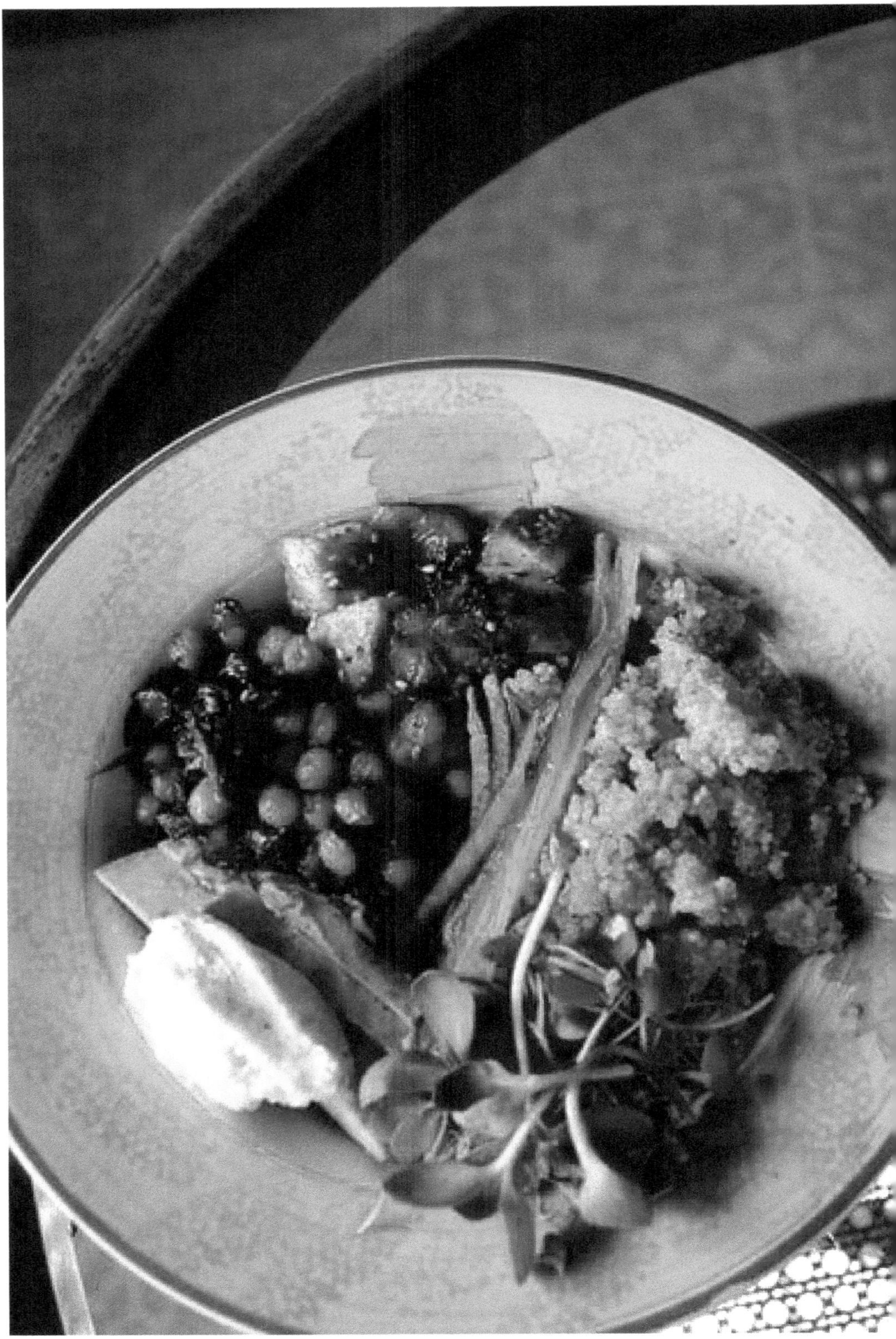

Spicy Vegetable Paella

8 Servings

Preparation time: 35 minutes

Ingredients

- 4 tbsps olive oil
- 4 medium carrots, sliced
- 2 celery stalk, sliced
- 2 medium yellow onions, chopped
- 2 medium red bell peppers, diced
- 6 garlic cloves, chopped
- 16 oz green peas
- 2 cups Spanish brown rice
- 2 (14.5-oz) can diced tomatoes
- 5 cups vegetable broth
- 1 tsp crushed red pepper
- 1 tsp ground fennel seed
- ½ tsp saffron
- 4 cups oyster mushrooms
- 2 cups asparagus, chopped

Directions

- Heat the oil in a pot over medium temperature.

- Put in some carrots, celery, onion, bell pepper, and garlic.

- Heat for 5 minutes until tender.

- Put in green peas, rice, tomatoes, broth, salt, red pepper, fennel seeds, and saffron.

- Heat for 20 minutes.

- Mix in mushrooms and asparagus. Cook covered another 10 minutes.

DESSERTS

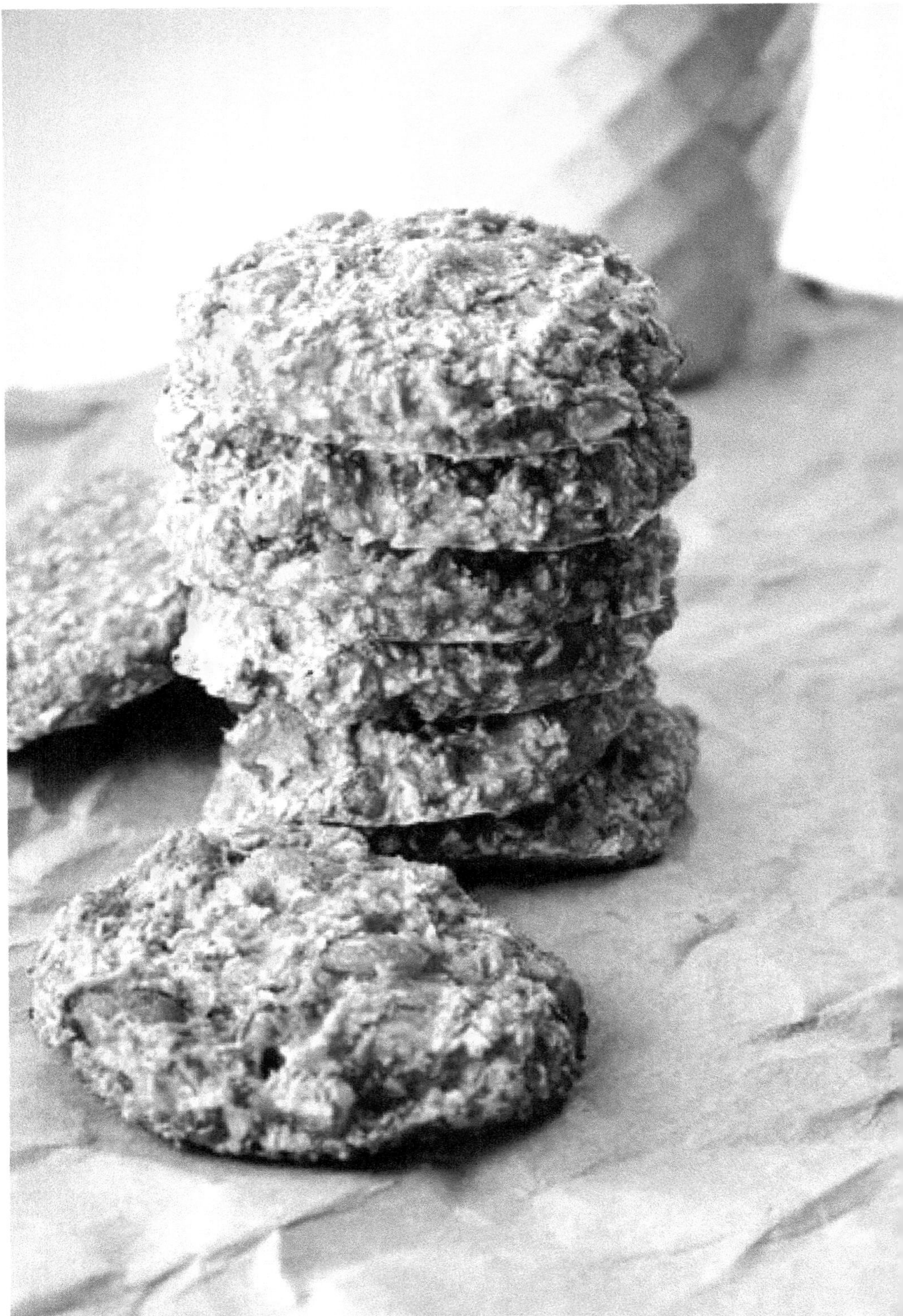

Raisin Oatmeal Biscuits

8 Servings

Preparation time: 20 minutes

Ingredients

- ½ cup plant butter
- 1 cup date sugar
- ¼ cup pineapple juice
- 1 cup whole-grain flour
- 1 tsp baking powder
- ½ tsp salt
- 1 tsp pure vanilla extract
- 1 cup old-fashioned oats
- ½ cup vegan chocolate chips
- ½ cup raisins

Directions

- Preheat oven to 370 F. Beat the butter and sugar in a bowl until creamy and fluffy. Pour in the juice and blend.

- Mix in flour, baking powder, salt, and vanilla. Stir in oats, chocolate chips, and raisins.

- Spread the dough on a baking sheet and bake for 15 minutes. Let completely cool on a rack.

Coconut & Chocolate Brownies

4 Servings

Preparation time: 40 minutes

Ingredients

- 1 cup whole-grain flour
- ½ cup unsweetened cocoa powder
- 1 tsp baking powder
- ½ tsp salt
- 1 cup pure date sugar
- ½ cup canola oil
- ¾ cup almond milk
- 1 tsp pure vanilla extract
- 1 tsp coconut extract
- ½ cup vegan chocolate chips
- ½ cup sweetened shredded coconut

Directions

- Preheat oven to 360 F. In a bowl, combine the flour, cocoa, baking powder, and salt.

- In another bowl, whisk the date sugar and oil until creamy. Add in almond milk, vanilla, and coconut extracts. Mix until smooth.

- Pour into the flour mixture and stir to combine. Fold in the coconut and chocolate chips.

- Pour the batter into a greased baking pan and bake for 35-40 minutes.

- Let cool before serving.

Cashew & Plum Cheesecake

4 Servings

Preparation time: 20 minutes

Ingredients

- 2/3 cup toasted rolled oats
- ¼ cup plant butter, melted
- 3 tbsps pure date sugar
- 6 oz cashew cream cheese
- ¼ cup oats milk
- ¼ cup just-boiled water
- 3 tsps agar agar powder
- 4 plums, cored and finely diced
- 2 tbsps toasted cashew, chopped

Directions

- Process the oats, butter, and date sugar in a blender until smooth. Pour the mixture into a greased 9-inch springform pan and press the mixture onto the bottom of the pan.

- Refrigerate for 30 minutes until firm while you make the filling.

- In a large bowl, using an electric mixer, whisk the cashew cream cheese until smooth.

- Beat in the oats milk. Mix the boiled water and agar agar powder until dissolved and whisk this mixture into the creamy mix. Fold in the plums.

- Remove the cake pan from the fridge and pour it in the plum mixture.

- Shake the pan to ensure smooth layering on top. Refrigerate for at least 3 hours.

- Take out the cake pan, release the cake, and garnish with the cashew nuts. Serve sliced.

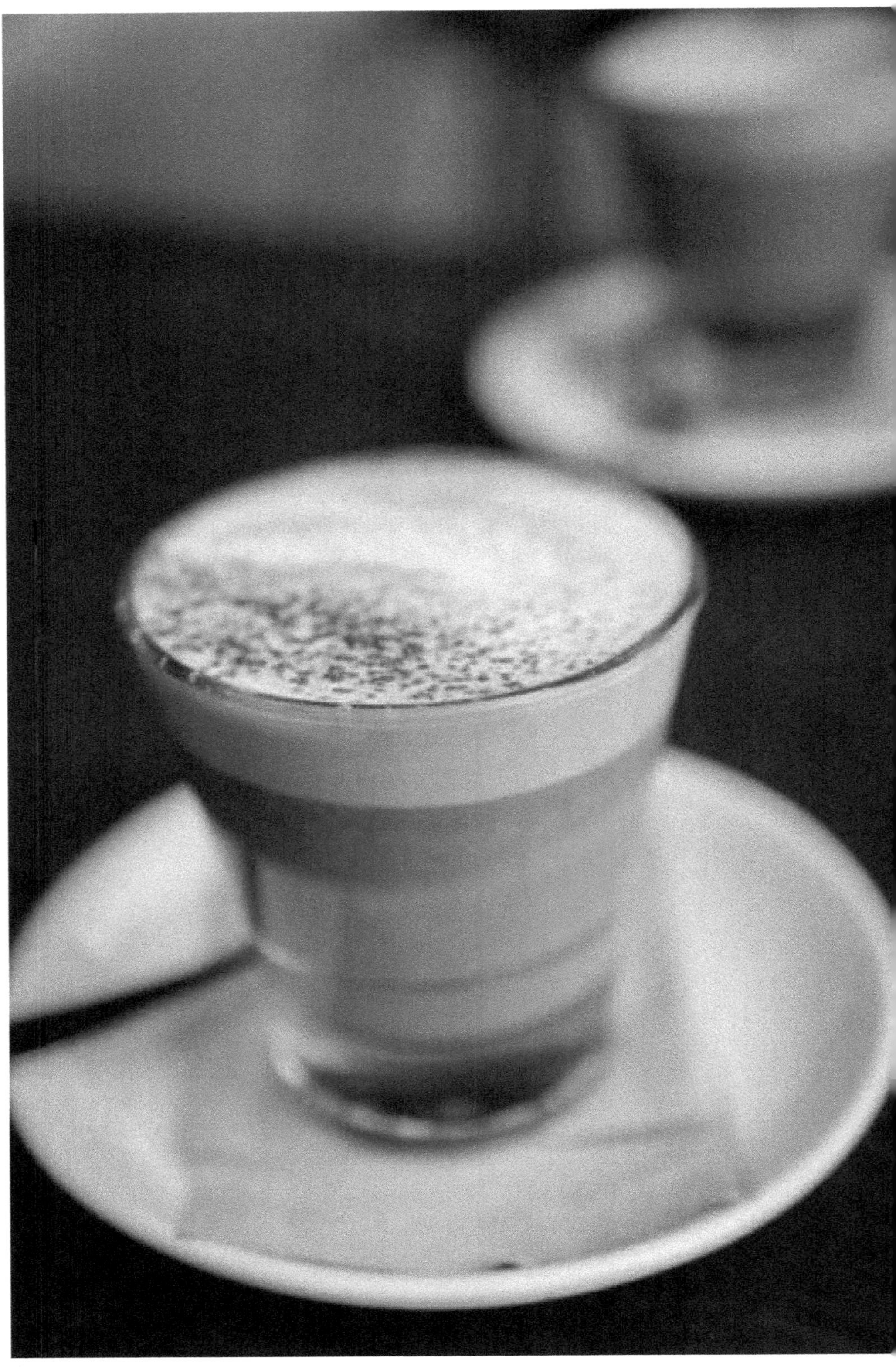

Peanut Chocolate Brownies

12 Servings

Preparation time: 45 minutes

Ingredients

- 1 ¾ cups whole-grain flour
- 1 tsp baking powder
- ½ tsp salt
- 1 tbsp ground nutmeg
- ½ tsp ground cinnamon
- 3 tbsps unsweetened cocoa powder
- ½ cup vegan chocolate chips
- ½ cup chopped peanuts
- ¼ cup canola oil
- ½ cup dark molasses ½ cup water
- ⅓ cup pure date sugar
- 2 tsps grated fresh ginger

Directions

- Preheat oven to 360 F.

- Combine the flour, baking powder, salt, nutmeg, cinnamon, and cocoa in a bowl. Add in chocolate chips and peanuts and stir. Set aside.

- In another bowl, mix the oil, molasses, water, sugar, and ginger. Pour into the flour mixture and stir to combine.

- Transfer to a greased baking pan and bake for 30-35 minutes. Let cool before slicing.

Chocolate Campanelle with Hazelnuts

4 Servings

Preparation time: 10 minutes

Ingredients

- ½ cup chopped toasted hazelnuts
- ¼ cup vegan chocolate pieces
- 8 oz campanelle pasta
- 3 tbsps vegan margarine
- ¼ cup maple syrup

Directions

- Pulse the hazelnuts and chocolate pieces in a food processor until crumbly. Set aside.

- Place the campanelle pasta in a pot with boiling salted water. Cook for 8-10 minutes until al dente, stirring often.

- Drain and back to the pot. Stir in almond butter and syrup and stir until the butter is melted.

- Remove to a plate and serve garnished with the chocolate-hazelnut mixture.

Poppy-Granola Balls with Chocolate

8 Servings

Preparation time: 25 minutes

Ingredients

- ½ cup granola
- ¼ cup pure date sugar
- ½ cup golden raisins
- ½ cup shelled sunflower seeds
- ¼ cup poppy seeds
- 1 ½ cups creamy almond butter
- 2 cups vegan chocolate chips

Directions

- Blend the granola, sugar, raisins, sunflower seeds, and poppy seeds in a food processor. Stir in the almond butter and pulse until a smooth dough is formed.

- Leave in the fridge overnight. Shape small balls out of the mixture. Set aside.

- Melt the chocolate in the microwave oven. Dip the balls into the melted chocolate and place on a baking sheet.

- Chill in the fridge for 30 minutes, until firm. Serve.

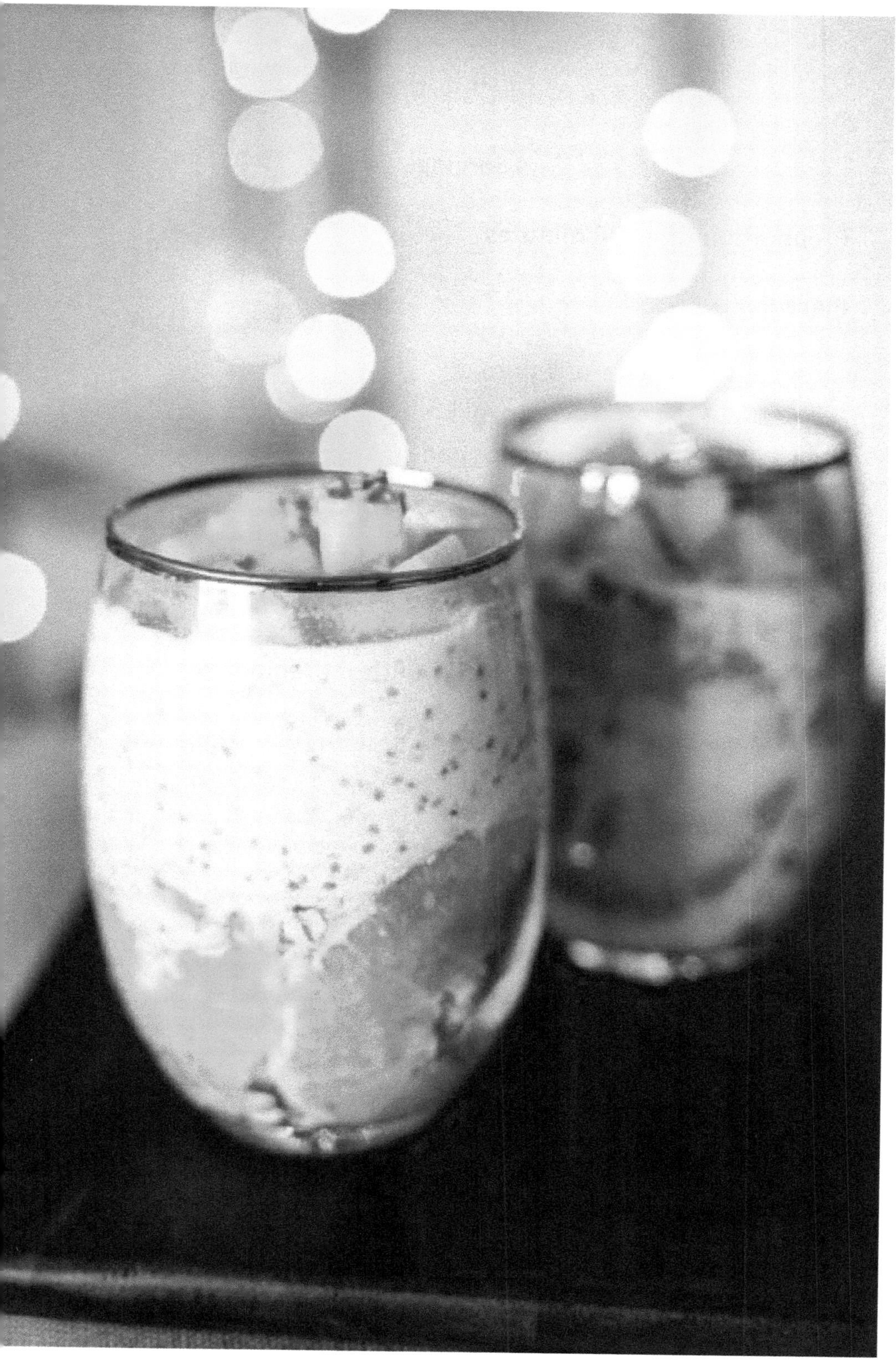

Coconut Chia Pudding

4 Servings

Preparation time: 30 minutes

Ingredients

- Zest and juice of 1 orange
- 1 (14-oz) can coconut milk
- 2 dates, pitted and chopped
- 1 tbsp chia seeds

Directions

- In a blender, put the orange juice, orange zest, coconut milk, dates, and chia seeds. Blitz until smooth.

- Transfer to a bowl and put it in the fridge for 20 minutes. Top with berries, whipped cream, or toasted coconut and serve.

Lightning Source UK Ltd.
Milton Keynes UK
UKHW020707130521
383649UK00005B/40

9 781802 854039